HEALTHY GUT & AUTOIMMUNE DIET 101

RECLAIM YOUR MICROBIOME HEALTH WITH 4 SIMPLE STEPS TO TAKE BACK CONTROL OF YOUR LONG-TERM HEALTH, MOOD AND WEIGHT

HOW TO HEAL YOUR MICROBIOME AND UNDERSTAND ITS INFLUENCE ON THE BRAIN

Written By
PURETURE, HHP

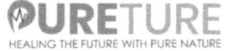

CONTENTS

Introduction   5

1. From the Brain in Our Gut to the Brain in Our Cranium   13
2. The Good, the Bad, and the Leaky Gut   23
3. 9 Warning Signs Your Gut Needs Healing   33
4. Top 5 Triggering Components Causing Poor Gut Health   56
5. Top 5 Foods to Naturally Heal the Gut   72
6. Top 5 Supplements to Naturally Heal the Gut   85
7. 4 Simple Steps to Heal Your Gut   94
8. 30-Day Plan to Heal Your Gut   108
9. Meal and Snack Options   115

Conclusion   121

© Copyright 2020 - All rights reserved.

It is not legal to reproduce, duplicate, or transmit any part of this document in either electronic means or in printed format. Recording of this publication is strictly prohibited and any storage of this document is not allowed unless with written permission from the publisher except for the use of brief quotations in a book review.

INTRODUCTION

Have you ever felt like you are not completely in control of the way you manage your lifestyle? As if you're not in control of the way you feel one moment to the next? You feel a sudden spring of energy as though you can just about tackle any task thrown at you, and then, somehow, in the next moment, you feel completely under the weather? What about when it comes to controlling the things you want to eat?

If you have ever felt like you were fighting yourself to keep control of your eating habits and your emotional states, that is because you are. We are not exactly fighting ourselves, but rather our microbiota, which comprises trillions of kinds of bacteria that influence our behavior. The more we feed the organisms that inhabit us, the more abundant they will become. Consequently, our cravings for what these organisms want will also increase.

Certain parts of us, mainly our microbiota, have been conditioned through a lifestyle that has been portrayed as "healthy." Modern life and—more importantly—modern hygiene have had their side effects on our behavior. Autoimmune diseases such as arthritis, Crohn's Disease, and irritable bowel syndrome are all common in our current era. These diseases have been directly associated with irregularities in the intestinal flora, which can cause permeability in the junctures of the intestinal lining (also known as Leaky Gut Syndrome). If you have a leaky gut, it means the intestinal lining is allowing unwanted particles and toxins to access your bloodstream, leading to inflammatory responses from your autoimmune system.

On the other hand, our mental health has been impacted as well. Depression and suicide rates are rising. In an age of comfort, where we don't have to go out to hunt our meals or pick our crops, you'd think we would be a lot happier. Unfortunately, statistics show this is not the case, and, in fact not hunting or growing our own crops plays a large role in the rise of these diseases. Comfort and hygiene have had their effects on the flora present in our gut. This is particularly alarming because the gut is considered our second brain, since it houses large amounts of neurons producing important neurotransmitters. These neurotransmitters are associated with reward systems which release serotonin and dopamine. These internal rewards incentivize and influence our behaviors.

Autoimmune diseases and mental health are treated in the traditional medical community, but they are not *cured*. As we know, treating an illness is a lot more profitable than curing it. There are different ways to alleviate a symptom, but if the root cause is not being addressed, relapse will occur. Having a label placed on you, like bipolar disorder, gives the perception that you have a lifelong condition that cannot be corrected, a condition that can only be treated with pharmaceuticals. Fortunately, this is not the case. In fact, change can occur in a matter of weeks. When referring to the gut, it is estimated that it takes about six weeks for the lining to be completely replaced by new cells. We should not allow ourselves to be categorized under an inescapable label or condition. Instead, we can take responsibility and control the way we take care of ourselves and our microbiota.

By now, you might be wondering who I am and how I know what I'm talking about. First, yes, my name is Pureture (think of pure with nature or future), and that is where Pureture Wellness's name came from, along with its slogan "Healing the Future with Pure Nature." As the founder of Pureture Wellness, a center for natural, holistic solutions to health and wellness, I can personally attest to the benefits of healing the gut for better brain function and an improved life overall.

Like you are probably feeling now, I was once a crazy person—literally. I was a fighter, both physically and mentally. I even tattooed myself with the phrase "fighting Irish." I was constantly agitating people and blaming them for my unsuccessful life. I took out my aggression on gym equipment by throwing heavy objects around; it was a way to numb my feelings. After many years of this unacceptable behavior, I finally realized I had some problems. I made the decision to throw away all of those man-made chemical supplements I had been using. Deep down, I knew and felt they were ruining my brain function, my mental state, my organs, and even though I had the body I wanted, they were also ruining me physically. The price I was paying for a nice-looking physique was simply too high. I was killing my body, my mind, and my soul with these poisonous chemicals. I knew I had to change ASAP!

My mood had cost me many friendships and romantic partners. As a result, I became extremely depressed, and the conventional medical community wanted to diagnose me with bipolar disorder. I refused that label, and I finally said, "Enough is enough!" I took responsibility for my own health and made huge changes, both inside and outside. At this point, I wanted nothing to do with pills and diagnoses, so I began to study. I worked with several mentors to begin applying healthy practices and transforming my life. Six years and one deep, intensive, healing journey later, I founded Pureture Wellness. My goal with this company is to help people like you implement the same healthy changes I made to achieve the physical and mental benefits of ridding your body of toxic chemicals.

One of our main goals at Pureture Wellness is to help people understand the connections between external (environment and nurture) and internal (microbiota, brain, and genetics) factors. In other words, we have a holistic approach to our methodology, which means we take into consideration the "whole" picture. Environmental factors, such as stress or how we nurture ourselves, will affect the way our microbiota is constituted, which will then affect our behavior through the influence of neurotransmitters in our gut.

We want you to provide yourself with an opportunity to change. At the very least, we can help you reflect upon your lifestyle, but in reality, it will do much more than that. When I say "we," I mean myself and the other holistic health coaches involved in our work here at Pureture Wellness. We are an organization whose mission is to provide people with access to information that will help them take control of their lives once and for all. This information will sometimes be in contrast to what mainstream media might have you believe.

We urge you to take this intensively healing journey. We are here to guide you through it and make it as simple and insightful as possible. I will be speaking to you from a theoretical and empirical background, since I too took this journey just like you are about to.

Truthfully, I had to endure quite a few harsh blows from life before I decided to take responsibility for myself and look to make a change. From losing friends and partners, to falling into a depression, I had taken a passive role when it came to my well-being. That's actually what the word "patient" implies. It assigns people a passive role and removes the active and responsible aspects a person should obtain when looking to improve their well-being. I was in "great shape" and trained at the gym regularly, I ate food considered healthy, and my exterior physical appearance was one many would covet. To say the least, it was quite a shock when I found out I was not leading a healthy lifestyle.

Evidence of the damage started manifesting in different ways. I was angry, confused, and often experienced brain fog. This led to being labeled with Bipolar Personality Disorder. I experienced hormonal imbalances occurring along with many digestive complications. Needless to say, this had a negative effect on my social interactions. These are aspects we don't normally associate with each other. They are factors that aren't as easily noticed as obesity, but which still have the capability of being life-ruining. It is a terrible experience to fall out of favor with loved ones due to an inability to control our own emotions. Worse, we rarely associate such issues in our interpersonal relations with what we choose to eat.

The first step is accepting and realizing there may be an issue. Once I accepted that my behavior was not serving me well, I took it upon myself to begin searching for a solution. After extensive research and experimenting, I came across likeminded people who had similar issues and had strived to look for solutions themselves. These people were my mentors and holistic health coaches who helped me realize how everything is interconnected. They opened my eyes to how my gut could be affecting my relationships, the chemical imbalances in my body, and even my levels of motivation. After this insight, my life started to turn around, and I began to find success in many of the areas that had been lacking.

As you can imagine, this is why I am so passionate about wanting to share this information with as many people as possible. It's important for us at Pureture Wellness to make this information easy to understand and the steps as simple as possible so other people can experience these changes themselves.

The best part is that we are here to provide you with the guidance needed to complete this process. We are holistic life coaches with more than a decade and—currently while writing this book—approximately fifteen years of research and experimenting in the field.

Remember, the symptoms you are experiencing aren't shackles you must carry throughout the rest of your life; there is a possibility for change. Awareness and commitment are all that is required. Commitment is soon followed by habit, making a new lifestyle even easier to follow. This has proven to be the case when it comes to having your brain/gut in the proper condition, as everything else will soon fall into place. First, we shall gain an understanding of the gut. It is my absolute hope and wish you enjoy this book and gain an incredible amount of knowledge.

Recommendation from the Pureture Wellness team:

We would like to make this journey you are about to embark on as smooth as possible. As with any journey, preparations need to be made, and there are tools fit for each pilgrimage. In our case, we require the Detox Goodies Toolkit, which is completely free. Not using these tools is like making a trip to a rainforest without insect repellant to protect yourself from mosquitoes. You can do it, but the experience won't be quite as seamless as it could have been. it can even be risky.

Please access the following link: https://www.pureture.com/detox-goodies/

In this link, you will find the following components:

- 20 Daily Detox Tips
- 15 Detox Tea Formulas
- 10 Detox Juices
- Master Shopping List: Healing and Detox Food

It may not yet be clear why these components are essential, but in further chapters, you will notice this information is required. When you begin the practical side of the work, you will understand. These tools are meant to alleviate some stress and obstacles that may show up along the way. For the time being, let's start by understanding the theory this practice is based on.

1

FROM THE BRAIN IN OUR GUT TO THE BRAIN IN OUR CRANIUM

WHAT ARE WE REFERRING TO WHEN WE SAY "GUT"?

By now, we have used the word "gut" several times. This refers to the section in the digestive system/gastrointestinal tract that extends from the pyloric sphincter of the stomach to the anus. This means the term "gut" does not include the stomach. This section between the stomach and the anus is divided in two main sections: the small intestine (or small bowel) and the large intestine (or colon/large bowel). Furthermore, the small intestine is divided itself into three more subsections: the duodenum, jejunum, and ileum.

To grasp the following terms we are about to introduce, let's go through the digestive process. Digestion is the process by which we break down complex molecules into simple molecules, either mechanically or enzymatically. The reason they are broken down, or digested, is so these simpler molecules may be absorbed and placed into the bloodstream where they are transported to the rest of the body (Ebneshsahidi, 2006). This process begins at the mouth where the food is chewed, then proceeds to the esophagus and finally the stomach. At this point, the food is churned and mixed with acid to be turned into chyme. Chyme is part gastric juices and part semi-digested food, which is then introduced into the small intestine.

The uppermost part of the small intestine is the duodenum. This is where the chyme goes next, and is also where most of our digestion occurs. The digestive process is carried out in the duodenum through the villi (see Figure 1), which are little sacks on the side of our intestinal walls. Their shape provides an increased surface area so they can catch molecules such as proteins, carbohydrates, and lipids. However, these protrusions have even smaller microscopic protrusions called microvilli, or brush border (see Figure 2), which also serve to catch more molecules and break them down even further (Ebneshsahidi, 2006). In other words, the fingers on our intestinal walls have even smaller little fingers themselves.

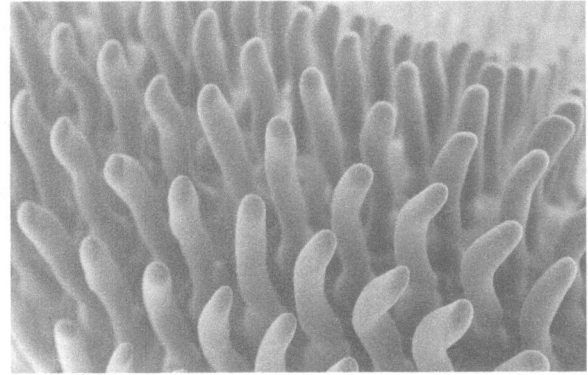

Fig. 1: 3D Villi Model.

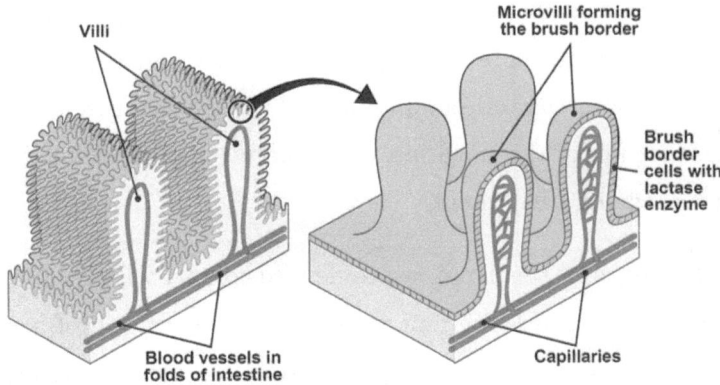

Fig. 2: Microvilli and Brush Border Enzymes.

Now that we have a clearer picture of what the villi and their microvilli look like, we can discuss the role of these pouches. Microvilli have specific types of enzymes attached to them that serve as catalysts during the process of breaking down these molecules. Each enzyme has its specific target, or match. Lactase, for example, is the enzyme that turns the disaccharide lactose into monosaccharides, splitting these into glucose and galactose. These simpler molecules are then processed by the enterocyte (intestinal absorptive cells) and transferred to the bloodstream. This process applies to all types of molecules, except for lipids, which have their own duct inside the enterocytes (Ebneshsahidi, 2006). This process of transferring the simple molecules into the bloodstream is called absorption.

To recap, we break down the molecules through digestion in order to facilitate the absorption process. After being digested in the duodenum, the chyme continues on to the jejunum and the ileum, where it is absorbed. While most absorption occurs in the jejunum, there are important nutrients absorbed in the ileum as well (Ebneshsahidi, 2006). The ileum is the bottom-most section of the small intestine, and we do absorb nutrients such as vitamin B12 there.

Following after the ileum, we come into contact with the colon. The colon is where we find the largest concentration of bacteria. These ecological systems of intestinal bacteria are referred to as microbiota. To gain some perspective, we have approximately one hundred thousand bacteria per gram of dry stool in the ileum, while in the colon we may find one trillion bacteria per gram. The amount of bacteria here provides us a clue as to what kind of activities are carried out in the colon. This is mainly where we receive assistance from our bacterial flora in the absorption and production of vitamins and minerals such as short-chain fatty acids, namely acetate, propionate, and butyrate. These products are referred to as metabolites, which play several beneficial roles in our defense against diabetes, obesity, autoimmune inflammation, and neurodegenerative diseases (Thursby & Juge, 2017).

MICROBIOTA AND MICROBIOME

The bacterial flora, or microbiota, of our gut includes fungi, bacteria, and archaea. A microbiome is the sum of all the genetic material in the gut, including both microbiota and their products, which we may refer to as metabolites. But where do these organisms come from?

Until recently, we thought the microbiota colonization process of a newborn would begin during labor. At this point, the infant would enter into contact with their mother's vaginal and cervical fluids, which are rich in microbial cells, and the child would be colonized.

However, Aagaard et al. (as cited in Dunn et al., 2017) mention that colonization may very well begin in utero. In fact, there may even already be existing microbiota in the placenta. Although they have been found in small quantities, further research needs to be made in order to understand the first stages of colonization. For the time being, however, the stance is that gut and vaginal microbes are the main source of microbial transference from mothers to infants (Nuyen-Ohayon, Neuman, & Koren as cited in Dunn et al., 2017). *Lactobacillus* is one of the predominant genera in the vaginal ecosystem which inhibits the growth of potentially pathogenic bacteria by increasing the acidity in the environment and competing for nutrients. This type of behavior is also found in the gut and serves as one of the reasons why we should keep certain strains of microbes healthy.

It is said that children born from cesarean are more likely to develop asthma/allergies (Black, Bhattacharya, Philip, Norman & Mclernon as cited in Dunn et al., 2017), inflammatory bowel disease (Kristensen & Hendriksen as cited in Dunn et al., 2017) and obesity (Bernardi et al. as cited in Dunn et al., 2017) than children born vaginally. Furthermore, there is also a correlation in children born through c-section and the likelihood of exhibiting traits associated with the autistic personality spectrum. The microbiome in a child born via cesarean is quite different to its mother's microbiome, as compared to a child born through the vaginal canal. A child born through c-section is influenced by skin and oral microbes, not to mention bacteria found in the operating room. This highlights the importance of controlling and maintaining the strains and diversity found in our microbiome. From the start, we can see that not being exposed to the appropriate amounts of bacteria can result in adverse effects to our health. In fact, antibiotics taken by a pregnant woman are a risk factor that may affect the diversity found in the microbiome. Prenatal conditions and factors are influential, but they are not life-defining either. After about six months, a person's microbiome starts to be defined more by the environment and what is consumed as nourishment, and less defined by the mother's microbiome (Dunn et al., 2017). However, like with many other developmental issues, there are critical stages of development that can have a larger influence in the long-term.

The mechanisms by which the bacteria in our gut affect the way we eat, which can lead us to obesity and other conditions, will be discussed in chapter 2. Before we dive into the relationship between microbiota and the brain, let's overview the makeup of the nervous system with which the microbiota is interacting.

THE SECOND BRAIN

The gut is often referred to as the second brain. This is largely due to the amount of neurons present in our intestinal tract that are relevant to our behavior. Our enteroendocrine cells are the main pathway to the vagus nerve, which is the main duct whereby electrochemical information is transferred from the gut to the brain. These are cells located on our brush border, which is another name for the microvilli located on our intestinal wall. These enteroendocrine cells communicate through hormonal messages and then synapse or connect to the vagus nerve. Specifically, the cells that synapse with nerves are called neuropod cells. These have the capacity of sensing and reacting to thermal, chemical, and mechanical stimuli, which may come from organic matter present in the gut, including microbes and their byproducts. Once these stimuli is received, the neuropod cells convert the information into small electrical impulses. Vagal neurons then carry these messages to the brain stem. The brain stem is in charge of communicating with the rest of the body, which only takes seconds at most, meaning that food in the gut will influence brain activity rather quickly, and the same goes for pathogens (Sharon et al., 2016).

We have decided to call our second brain the enteric nervous system. It is autonomous from our central nervous system, and can carry out gastrointestinal functions on its own, even if communication is cut off from the brain. This nervous system is made of layers of neurons spread out all across our gut, reaching the end of the large intestine. Important neurotransmitters are both produced and stored in the gut, inside specialized cells called enterochromaffin cells. In fact, ninety-five percent of the serotonin, popularly known as the "happiness hormone," in our bodies is both produced and stored here. The way we synthesize serotonin is through compounds received via the food we consume. Aside from this, our microbiota can stimulate or inhibit the production of serotonin. To be precise, sixty percent of the serotonin produced in our gut is due to microbial stimulation (Sharon et al., 2016). Low levels of serotonin are associated with depression, indicating that serotonin plays a large role in our emotional equilibrium.

The first piece of evidence linking our microbiota to brain function is provided by germ-free mice. Mice which were completely isolated from microbes—sterile, in other words—displayed increased risk-taking behaviors and hyperactivity while also exhibiting memory and learning deficits as compared to specific pathogen-free mice (Clarke et al., 2013; Gareau et al., 2011; Heijtz et al., 2011; Neufeld et al., 2011 as cited in Sharon et al., 2016). The specific pathogen mice, as implied by their name, are generally healthy and seemingly balanced. Another example is provided by Buffington (as cited in Sharon et al., 2016) by stating that administering mice with a high-fat diet during pregnancy was enough to lower the *Lactobacilli* population of bacteria in their gut, consequently leading to antisocial behavioral patterns in their offspring. These behaviors could be reversed at a later time by reintroducing *Lactobacillus* bacteria back into their microbiota. This clearly shows a correlation between behavioral patterns and the biodiversity of our intestinal flora. The absence of microbiota in the first case leads to maladaptive behavior. In the second case, we have a diminished amount of beneficial microbiota in a mother leading to the same result of adverse behavior patterns in subsequent offspring.

Just like any other ecosystem, your microbiota is also put to the Darwinian test of survival of the fittest. Also like any other biological environment, there is a certain level of balance required for sustainability. Each colony of bacteria is fighting for control of your gut, and consequently your behavior. Like many wars, external factors may influence the outcome. External factors in our case are generally food or environmental stimuli that we expose ourselves to. We do have a horse in this race, though. It is, as we shall explore, in our best interest for us to tip the scale in favor of certain organisms far more beneficial to our well-being. We have reached a state of endosymbiosis with some of these organisms, which means we have developed together with these organisms to the point where we need our microbiota as much as they need us.

CHAPTER SUMMARY

In this chapter, we've discussed the brain and the second brain known as the gut. Specifically, we've covered the following topics:

- The digestive system/gastrointestinal tract with illustrations of their makeup and the process of breaking down complex molecules
- The microbiota vs. microbiome and why they are important to understand
- The second brain and its relation to the nervous system

In the next chapter, you will learn about good bacteria, bad bacteria and Leaky Gut Syndrome.

2

THE GOOD, THE BAD, AND THE LEAKY GUT

A BRIEF OVERVIEW OF THE HISTORY OF DISEASE

Our perception of where disease comes from has has changed over the last couple centuries due to technological advancement. We shall explore the relationship between a healthy microbiome and different propensities to disease, as well as the relationship between microbiota, what we consume, and our environment.

The theory about microorganisms as the cause of disease originated in the nineteenth century (Shumsky, N., 1998). Prior to this theory, it was believed that miasma was the cause for disease instead. There have been references to the concept of miasma since Ancient Greece. The most recent conception of miasma is that of nature's production of pestilent air, often found in swamps and forests. Along with this conception came the thought that all man-made chemicals were clean and could rid us of the pestilence and disease that nature brought about.

This concept of miasma was then discarded by the concept of germs, which are microscopic organisms that reside everywhere and were the new culprits of disease. However, the influence from the miasma theory remains. As we will come to see, not all microorganisms are pathogenic (disease-causing microorganisms). In fact, we require a healthy diversity of microorganisms to function optimally. The problem lies in the fact that this idea has not yet been embedded into our modern lifestyle. Society remains at war with germs.

This war against germs, and this conception of germs causing disease, is true to a certain degree. The fluoride and chlorine in our water are not all evil; in fact, they are keeping us from succumbing to disease-producing pathogens such as *cholerae*, which was commonplace not too long ago. Entire families could be wiped out due to pathogenic infections. However, our cleansing chemicals do betray us. The hygiene hypothesis states that, due to smaller family sizes and artificially cleaner environments, people come in less contact with childhood diseases (Smith, Bloomfield, & Rook, 2012). To support this theory, which mentions that we may be a bit "too clean" for our own good, Smith et al. (2012) expresses that there may be a correlation between the increased standards of cleanliness and the rising amount of allergic disorders, not to mention autoimmune diseases, type 1 diabetes, and irritable bowel syndrome. We would imagine that these types of diseases would decrease with our increasing levels of hygiene, but it doesn't seem to be the case. It is great that we have found a way to fight off pathogens, but excessive cleanliness has also taken a toll on our necessary microorganisms.

Let's think back to the germ-free mice we talked about. The sterile ones did show cognitive deficiencies, giving us a clue as to how important microorganisms are to our normal brain functions. Keeping that in mind, ask yourself what alcohol is designed for? One of its most popular uses is to combat bacteria. What do you think happens when you drink it? It won't discriminate the good bacteria from the bad. The same goes for chlorine in water, and the fluoride in your toothpaste. Antibiotics, while they are necessary, don't do a great job at discriminating either. One final factor to take into consideration is stress, which is chemically expressed through the hormone cortisol. There has been a correlation drawn between higher levels of cortisol leading to lower levels of *lactobacillus* in our gut (Smith, Bloomfield, & Rook, 2012). *Lactobacillus* is one of the good guys, which will be reviewed in detail. We shall take a look at why it is so important to support our good bacteria, or at least to keep a reasonable balance so dysbiosis does not occur. Dysbiosis is the term that refers to a state of microbial imbalance or impairment.

LEAKY GUT SYNDROME

Many factors, including stress, antibiotics, hygiene, and an improper diet, can change or destroy the composition of our microflora. This imbalance and destruction of probiotics (benevolent bacteria) can allow the overgrowth of more opportunistic entities. One we would like to specifically point out is the fungi of the *Candida albicans* strain. Studies have shown a relationship between this strain of fungus in our gut and an increase of our intestinal permeability. This fungus installs roots in the intestinal lining called hyphae, which leads to holes by which toxins, undigested foods, and other microorganisms can pass through into the bloodstream, consequently being transported to the rest of the body. This rupture of the tight junctions held in the intestinal lining is called Leaky Gut Syndrome. After the tiny openings have been created by the hyphae, these roots then continue to grow and push apart the junctions holding our intestinal lining together. When this happens, our body's immune responses fire, and we start creating antibodies. We perceive these stages of the process through symptoms such as food allergies and inflammatory or autoimmune responses (Pushpanathan, 2016).

As serious as all this sounds, Leaky Gut Syndrome isn't a main focus for the medical institution, particularly since they don't have an easy way of diagnosing and testing for it. As a result, it is a frequently overlooked condition . In fact, some physicians might choose to simply treat the symptoms because the root cause is somewhat unknown. People experiencing conditions such as fibromyalgia, depression, or arthritis are aware of how vague a doctor can be about the cause of their illness. More research has begun to point to the fact that the way we eat may be playing a much larger and direct role in these conditions of typically unknown origin. Unfortunately, a lot of the pain medication prescribed for this disease just worsens the state of the microbiome. They may make you feel better for some time, but in the long-run, the damage accumulates. The fact that the the medical industry does not seriously consider the microbiome will lead to many more cases of undiagnosed conditions, including a possible epidemic of depression and autoimmune diseases (Pushpanathan, 2016). In chapter 3, we will take a look at more specific interactions between Leaky Gut Syndrome and other conditions which plague our era.

PROBIOTICS & PATHOGENS

Probiotics are normal, harmless bacteria that provide health benefits. If taken in the right doses, these can lead to nutritional benefits by helping populate our gut with the bacteria responsible for facilitating the absorption process. *Lactobacillus* and *Bifidobacterium* are strains that belong in this category. It is necessary to regularly consume food which contains or nourishes these strains in order to keep a healthy, balanced microbiome. Yogurt might come to mind when you hear the term probiotics; unfortunately, this type of food isn't as beneficial as mainstream media would have you believe. You obtain minimal amounts of the organisms while obtaining high amounts of refined sugars, which aid other less-beneficial bacteria in your microbiome. Aside from providing a balanced ecosystem, consuming foods with probiotics will prevent the colonization of pathogens and increase the vitamin availability in our body. As Rolhion and Chassaing mention, "By consuming common limited resources, the gut microbiota induces the starvation of competing pathogens, this is called colonization resistance" (2016, p.2). Some microorganisms even metabolize harmful toxins into less harmful components in our gut, acting as a filter of sorts (Abatenh, et al., 2018).

Lactobacillus and *Bifidobacterium* are known for their capacity to rule out and prevent pathogens from growing. There are quite a few other strains of probiotics (see Table 1), but these are the most popular. These probiotics protect us by changing the pH or acid/base levels in our gut. They lower the pH via probiotic-produced organic acids called bacteriocins, creating an antagonistic environment where food-spawned pathogens may not thrive. That is at least one way *Lactobacilli* protects us.

We also mentioned that the microbiota in our colon produce butyrate, which is used to combat *Salmonella* pathogens commonly originating from poultry. *C. difficile* is one of the more popular disease-causing bacteria, which is known for diarrhea and nausea. *C. difficile* infections can be life-threatening in the later stages, but we have discovered we are able to combat *C. difficile* by introducing its competitor, *Bacteroides thuringiensis,* to our microbiome. One of the methods to do this is by submitting a healthy person's fecal matter into a patient infected with *C. diff.* The success rate related to this treatment method is quite high but is only necessary in severe cases where the infection is advanced.

Aside from making an antagonistic environment for pathogens, probiotics can also create a physical/chemical barrier that doesn't allow certain pathogens to roam free in our gut. This is called the microbial barrier. If these acts of heroism aren't enough to convince you they are the good guys, probiotics are also known to have a large amount of control over our autoimmune responses. They do this by interacting with the enteric nervous system through electrochemical messages (Abatenh, et al., 2018).

In an effort to summarize the role probiotics take in our health, consider the three following statements. Probiotics play a large role in the healthy functioning of the intestinal immune system. They enhance nutrient acquisition by improving the metabolic processes of the gut. Finally, probiotics provide colonization resistance from endogenous and exogenous pathogens through antagonistic environment control. For these reasons, we must help tip the scales of this battle to ensure our probiotic population is healthy and diverse. The first step to change is awareness (Rolhion & Chassaing, 2016).

List of probiotic species	Group of Microbes
Lactobacillus sacidophilus, Lactobacillus bulgaricus, Lactobacillus casei, Lactobacillus fermentum, Lactobacillus lactis, Lactobacillus acidophilus, Lactobacillus pariscasei, L. rhamnosus, L. delbrueckii subsp. bulgaricus, L. brevis, L. johnsonii, Lactobacillus plantarum, Lactobacillus salivarius, Lactobacillus fermentum, Lactobacillus kefir	Lactic acid producing bacteria
Enterococcus faecalis, Enterococcus faecium, Escherichia coli Nissle, Streptococcus thermophiles, Propinobacterium	Non lactic acid producing bacteria
Bifidobacterium adolescentis, Bifidobacterium bifidum, Bifidobacterium breve, Bifidobacterium lactis, Bifidobacterium longum, Bifidobacterium infantis, B. animalis subsp animalis, B. animalis subsp lactis, B. bifidum	Bifidobacterium species
Saccharomyces boulardii	Nonpathogenic yeast
Coccobacillus, Lactobacillus, Streptococcus, Leuconostoc, Lactococcus lactis subsp. Lactis, Pediococcus, Propionibacterium, Enterococcus, Enterococcus durans, Bifidobacterium, Bacillus, Bacillus coagulans, Bacillus subtilis, Saccharomyces cerevisiae, Candida pintolopesii, Aspergillus niger, A. oryzae, Bacillus lichenformis, B. cereus var. toyoi, B. clausii, B. coagulans, B. laterosporus, B. pumilus, B. racemilacticus, Streptococcu sthermophiles	Non spore forming

Table 1: List of Probiotic Species.

Going back to our less than fortunate germ-free mice, it was evidenced that exposing these mice to exogenous pathogens resulted in much larger infections. The fact that they didn't have any sort of microbial protection to keep the pathogens away from the villi, and therefore the bloodstream, had catastrophic effects. It is important to remember that even if dysbiosis is reached, we can still correct our microbiome and regain equilibrium. Even if Leaky Gut Syndrome were is present, studies show that providing multi-strain probiotics containing numerous strains of *Lactobacilli* can correct this condition since *Lactobacillus* and butyrate both play a large role in intestinal lining integrity.

Two main ways that pathogens gain the upper hand in our ecosystem is through changes in our internal pH and the type of food available to our microbiota. Certain types of carbohydrates that are more difficult to digest will lead to increased microbial fermentation. The increase of gases and microbial products then stimulate our villi to set off local inflammation, which causes intestinal permeability, or leaky gut. Once again, *C. difficile* is one of the main culprits, as it can become predominant and infect us through a change in the pH levels of our stomach. Our stomach is our first point of defense against many types of pathogens. Most are killed off by the stomach acid, but when stomach acid levels decrease *C. diff* can begin to propagate. *C. diff* causes symptoms such as diarrhea, nausea, and intestinal inflammation, the latter of which causes leaky gut. When the conditions are right, such as a high animal protein (meat and dairy) and low-fiber diet, *C. diff* can thrive. This reduces the number of beneficial bacteria and even invites other harmful bacteria such as *Candida* to take over. The focal point to take away here would be that studies show excess animal protein can stimulate the growth of pathogens such as *C. difficile*. At the same time, a lack of fiber in our diet will make it so that our microbiota cannot compete with exogenous pathogens. Next, we will take a look at the specific effects pathogens may have on our body when our gut is in a state of dysbiosis.

CHAPTER SUMMARY

In this chapter, we discussed the following topics:

- A brief overview of the history of disease

- Leaky Gut Syndrome and the disconnect with the medical institutions
- Probiotics and pathogens

In the next chapter, you will learn about the top warning signs from your body as an indication that your gut needs healing.

3

9 WARNING SIGNS YOUR GUT NEEDS HEALING

1. Food Sensitivities
2. Gas and Bloating
3. Irritable Bowel Diseases
4. Autoimmune Diseases
5. Malabsorption: Nutritional Deficiencies
6. Thyroids and Energy Production
7. Emotional Disturbances
8. Behavioral Disturbances: Food Preferences
9. Obesity

Now that we understand the underlying mechanisms that provide us with a self-sustaining microbial ecosystem, it becomes imperative for us to distinguish when we might be falling out of balance and into dysbiosis. In its initial stages, dysbiosis isn't necessarily life threatening. However, we should be alert to subtler symptoms as well. We will be able to notice there is a relationship between many of the warning signs, and that some may lead to others, possibly exacerbating each other. This is mainly due to the interconnectedness we can see in our body. We must look at the complete picture and understand the relationships created between the different parts. Let's discuss what it is we are looking for when we want to be aware of irregularities in our own microbial equilibrium.

1. FOOD SENSITIVITIES OR ALLERGIES

Food allergies are on the rise in our society, with about a fifty percent increase since 1997. Recent studies show that every 1 in 15 to 1 in 20 adults in the US and Canada suffer from a type of food allergy (Savage & Johns as cited in Benede et al., 2016). The number is much higher in Australia, with 1 in 10 being the prevalence. Further research has shed light on some factors leading to the origin of these allergies, supporting the idea that our modern lifestyle is too clean. The chemicals in our water, along with the excessive use of antibiotics, are the aspects of modern life that the hygiene hypothesis criticizes. In the experiment done on germ-free mice where their intestinal flora was destroyed through antibiotics, an allergy to peanuts arose, similar to that of children. After introducing microbial strains present in a healthy mice's microbiome, the allergy to peanuts was cured.

Further statistical analysis shows that children with older siblings or pets in their home are less likely to develop food allergies. This has to do with the amount of exposure children have to different microbial flora. The first three years of life are the most critical in this sense. This is contrary to our instincts; we feel that we are keeping our children safe by keeping them far away from germs. However, if a child is not exposed to a healthy diversity of microbes and colonized during the first three years of their life, it can have profound effects on their long-term health. This was tested on piglets, and the results were positive, verifying the correlation between pet germs and food allergies (Schmidt et al., as cited in Benede et al., 2016). Another piece of evidence shows that brushing pet dust on germ-free mice has served as a protective measure against asthma (Fujimura et al., as cited in Benede et al., 2016). This could help us reflect upon the relationship we have with nature, including how we are part of our environment and should not try to segregate ourselves artificially. This is mainly because our environment needs us as much as we need it. Having a holistic point of view is necessary to be able to see all the factors that play a role in our well-being, in seeing the interconnectedness that is truly necessary for a self-sustaining system such as our body and our planet.

Environmental exposure to microbes through pets and siblings is ideal, but we are often exposed through what we eat. I can attest from personal experience that the symptoms from food allergies can be reversed by balancing our bacterial flora.

Allergic symptoms will be perceived when the intestinal lining in our gut is compromised. This makes it so the cells on our microvilli can't be so selective and can allow protein molecules that have not been broken down by digestion to pass through. Once these irregular molecules are absorbed into the bloodstream, our bodies fire an immune response, treating the molecules as foreign bodies. This consequently leads to inflammation, which further damages the junction on the intestinal lining, leading to more sensitivity to the food. It is a cycle: Leaky gut can stimulate food allergies, and food allergies make your leaky gut even leakier (Benede et al., 2016). Your food allergy may have first occurred due to an imbalance in bacterial flora. Candida are known to be a doorway to food allergies by opening up small holes with their roots (hyphae).

I unknowingly suffered from certain subtle intolerances myself, such as an unwarranted headache that might come about for no apparent reason, or waking up one day lethargic and having difficulty focusing. I would perceive these symptoms as part of my body's normal functioning. Then I did some extensive research coupled together with the method I am going to provide to you. I was able to find out which types of gluten, dairy, and meat were causing which symptoms. I came to find out that certain types of gluten would add water weight and cause a puffy look, specifically around my eyes and ankle joints. If you happen to be suffering from this type of symptom, it is not too late to begin changing the composition of your intestinal flora. Whether you have had allergies since you were a child, or you are now developing sensitivities as an adult, it is in your best interest to strengthen the junctures of your intestinal lining.

2. GAS & BLOATING

Now, let's keep in mind that flatulence is a normal function of our body, and we should only be seeing this as a bad sign if we feel it has become excessive. Gas may be one of the more subtle signs our body gives us when trying to tell us that something is wrong. There are a variety of reasons why a person may be experiencing gas or bloating. It might seem hard to narrow down the culprit, but the more information you can gather about your reactions to different foods and circumstances, the better idea you will have as to what triggers your symptoms.

Most often, gas is caused by inadequate protein digestion or an inability to break down carbohydrates and sugars. Even this lack of digestion is influenced by bacterial flora. Deficiency in digestion is often caused by excess levels of *H. pylori*. These microbes will change your stomach's pH level and make it less acidic. This will cause several complications, including inadequate digestion, allowing microbes and molecules that would normally be dealt with in the stomach to flow downstream into the gut. Once these microbes find their way to the gut, we will be looking at a possible dysbiosis if certain strains start to overpopulate the small intestine. On the other hand, the arrival of molecules that should have been broken down will lead to an abundance of certain types of foods that may tilt the scale towards our less beneficial microbiota. So, no matter which way we put it, microflora will play a large role in gas and bloating.

Gas is mainly produced through bacterial fermentation. This happens when we consume unabsorbed or non-absorbable sugars (i.e., alcohol), and carbs which may be difficult to digest (i.e., dairy and baked beans). Intolerance to certain carbs and proteins such as dairy and eggs are common causes for excessive gas, which leads to bloating. In the case of dairy products, a lack of lactase enzymes will make it so lactose (protein in milk) is carried to the colon in its complete state. In the colon, there are microbes that can digest these proteins into methane. This is what leads to the excess amounts of gas evidenced in people suffering from lactose intolerance. Balancing your pH will create an environment where your microbiota can thrive in a balanced manner, allowing for easier digestion. There are some foods that should be avoided as much as possible, and we will get into that in the following chapter.

3. IRRITABLE BOWEL DISEASES

Irritable Bowel Disease (IBD) is an umbrella term that describes states of intestinal irritability, causing inflammation. Ulcerative Colitis, for example, is described as inflammation in the inner-most region of our colon's lining. In severe cases, it leads to sores called ulcers. Crohn's Disease is described more as general inflammation in the whole intestinal lining. The pathogenesis (origin of the disease) is unknown. However, as we already know from the studies we have reviewed, the health of our intestinal lining is dependent on microbiota balance. In fact, in patients suffering from IBDs, certain overgrowth of microbial strains has been evidenced over others, such as *Candida albicans*, for example (Zuo & Siew, 2018). Common symptoms to look out for are chronic diarrhea, loss of appetite, unintended loss of weight, abdominal cramps, or blood in your stool.

The most common of symptoms is diarrhea. A reason why we might have acute diarrhea is because of a viral infection that can last from a couple of days to a couple of weeks. Bacterial infections can last longer, especially if the intestinal lining is damaged in the process. They can be less severe and less noticeable than viral infections. Damage to our intestinal lining itself can cause diarrhea by not allowing our brush border to absorb minerals and sugars appropriately. If we allow certain sugars, proteins, and minerals to remain abundant in our colon by not absorbing them, we will create the right conditions for pathogenic bacteria to thrive. This may lead to possible damage to the intestinal lining. When inflammation damages our intestinal lining, our ability to absorb salts and sugars decreases, leading to further diarrhea. Chronic diarrhea must be dealt with, or else it can turn into an IBD through repeatedly damaging the intestinal lining and causing an imbalance in the microflora (Zuo & Siew, 2018).

In general, diarrhea caused by viral infections does not necessarily cause inflammation. Since it does not cause inflammation, it is not damaging the intestinal lining. Diarrhea caused by bacteria is a whole other story, as this type does cause inflammation and destroys the intestinal lining, causing a leaky gut. The problem with this type of diarrhea is that it can persist and become chronic, since the inflammation itself causes further diarrhea due to the inability to absorb certain molecules in its damaged state. These types of infections have been fought off through hygiene, however. Even in the United States, 75,000 people are infected by *E. coli* and *C. difficile* every year, so this type of diarrhea is by no means a thing of the past (Hodges & Gill, 2010). As we saw with the germ-free mice, if you have your microbial barrier intact, your microbiota can help you fight off these types of long-lasting infections. We are not necessarily talking about diarrhea to the point where you are becoming dehydrated and can't walk. It may just be that you have it every other day for no apparent reason. Perhaps your stools are softer than they used to be. These are all signs that can be addressed before things get worse. Recovering the balance in our microflora and consequently repairing our intestinal lining will impoverish the living conditions for pathogens such as those of the *Candida, E. coli,* and *C. difficile* strains, all of which are associated with IBDs (Zuo & Siew, 2018).

4. AUTOIMMUNE DISEASES

In this category, we will find diseases such as fibromyalgia, rheumatoid arthritis, and type 1 diabetes. The root cause for these diseases still remains a mystery to the medical establishment. However, recent research is paying closer attention to our feeding patterns. This field of microbiotic research is fairly new; technological advancements have been occurring from 2002 and onward. In previous years, we could only examine cultured or cultivated microorganisms and not so much the organisms in their natural environment. This is the reason why so many studies are being conducted these days. The increase in research related to our microbiota will hopefully bring about new types of treatments and preventive medicine. Treatments are already being developed, and the scientific community is still working hard to support this shift in the way we perceive our health.

Eating excessive gluten, over-processed foods, excessive sugar, and even too much animal protein will eventually all cause a leaky gut. Once these food options are consumed for a prolonged period of time, they start triggering our autoimmune system. This leads to increased intestinal permeability. Autoimmune diseases are caused by the immune system losing the ability to differentiate proteins belonging to the body with the proteins belonging to a foreign invader (like bacterial infections, viruses, undigested food, gut cell components, or parasites). Symptoms are caused by a buildup of damage to cells, tissues, and/or organs in the body—damage caused by our immune system attacking those cells.

When it comes to type 1 diabetes, it is well-known that there can be a genetic predisposition to the disease. On the other hand, external factors have been reported as associations to its root cause. One factor found is that the consumption of dairy during early stages of life leads to a higher propensity to the disease. This shows the type of impact our diet has on the immune system, since type 1 diabetes is caused by an autoimmune response that destroys B cells. Further studies display a difference between the microflora found in people positive for type 1 diabetes as compared to people without the condition. The difference was marked by the ratio by which *Firmicutes* and *Bacteroidetes* strains were present (Pashou et al., 2018).

The cause of fibromyalgia, just like type 1 diabetes, also eludes us. In spite of this, research has shown that about seventy percent of people diagnosed with fibromyalgia also fit the criteria for Leaky Gut Syndrome. Unfortunately, Leaky Gut Syndrome magnifies the symptoms experienced in fibromyalgia, symptoms such as generalized pain and chronic fatigue. The symptoms are intensified through the persistent activation of our immune system by the molecules that slip into our bloodstream via our intestinal lining. Toxins coming through the permeable gut lining are transported all across the body to cause chronic inflammation everywhere as the body rejects these molecules that are not supposed to be there. Inflammation magnifies any injuries a person might have had in the past through increased sensitivity in our pain fibers localized at our joints, for example. These are factors which explain and maybe, in some cases, even cause the pain felt in fibromyalgia (Erdrich et al., 2020).

Addressing the chronic fatigue felt by people with fibromyalgia, part of the reason people describe "brain-fog" or a general slowness as a part of their symptoms is due to the pain fibers firing off constantly. This constant unnecessary activation of the immune system wears the brain out. We are using up our energy unnecessarily by communicating these pain signals to our brain. On top of this, our brain is also being trained and conditioned to detect pain through repetitive signaling, which makes it even more sensitive to any pain being experienced. Another reason people with fibromyalgia experience fatigue when they have a leaky gut is because they also have dysbiosis. This dysbiosis is specifically located in their small intestine and is called Small Intestine Bacterial Overgrowth, or SIBO for short. SIBO occurs when the plethora of bacteria that live in our colon start moving up into the small intestine. The small intestine is where most of our absorption occurs. When bacteria start to rise up to the small intestine, it makes us have to compete for nutrients with the bacteria that have found a new home there. This, of course, depletes our energy production. If microbiota health is important, it is even more so for people who suffer from fibromyalgia (Erdrich et al., 2020).

Arthritis is no exception to the pattern we have been following. All three diseases have unknown origins, yet clinical and experimental data have been associating these conditions with our gut health. Even if gut microorganisms were not the cause, the evidence shows that having a leaky gut magnifies the symptoms felt in these conditions. It's not all bad news, though; through the administration of probiotics there has been significant changes as to how the diseases progress. One of the ways we know that leaky gut has a role to play in arthritis is because bacterial cell wall components are found in the victim's joints, the same components present in the gut lining. Luckily, these situations are not as irreversible as some might think.

5. MALABSORPTION: NUTRITIONAL DEFICIENCIES

To this point, it is fairly clear that one of the main roles of our small intestine is to absorb nutrients. It does this through its permeability. We have been talking about intestinal permeability or Leaky Gut Syndrome as an issue. It is an issue when it becomes excessively permeable. This is what allows us to selectively absorb our nutrients into the bloodstream. The key word here is "selectively." When we lose the capacity to select what goes into our bloodstream, that is when we come across a leaky gut. Thankfully, due to the amount of different organisms our gut has to interact with, the sensors located in our gut can discriminate between good bacteria and pathogens, and likewise between nutrients and toxins.

Two main ways that malabsorption may occur are through faulty digestive processes and Small Intestine Bacterial Overgrowth. As we have mentioned, in the first case we would not be able to absorb our nutrients if they are not first broken down (Ghosh, 2010). This leads to whole molecules ending up in our colon and being metabolized by our colon's bacteria instead of being absorbed. The second scenario has been discussed as well. If bacteria that are supposed to stay in our colon rise up to our small intestine, they will compete with us for our nutrients. This leads to conditions such as anemia. On top of the fact that we are receiving a decreased amount of nutrients, we do perceive a loss of appetite in certain scenarios associated to SIBO. If these different warning signs may seem related, it is because they are. What we would be looking out for here is primarily less energy production and loss of appetite as possible indicators. These two have consequences of their own that may lead to emotional disturbances.

6. THYROIDS & ENERGY PRODUCTION

A lot of us may have heard the term thyroid, but we may not be aware of just how large of a role this gland plays in our well-being. We may begin by mentioning the mitochondria. Mitochondria could be viewed as the engines inside each and every one of the living cells in our body. They actually have their own

DNA and used to be their own species at some point in evolutionary history. Through the passage of time, these organisms have become a part of us through a process called endosymbiosis. As a result, mitochondria provide us with usable energy called ATP. These cells, however, will not produce this energy unless they are told to do so. This is where our thyroids come in. This gland pumps out a hormone called T3, which is then transported all over our body and used to signal mitochondria to produce ATP. This is the energy of life, and it is what we use to carry out any task, from a simple muscular movement to creating a new cell in our body. Both ATP and T3 are essential for our daily functioning.

For our thyroids to produce T3, it is necessary for them to receive a healthy amount of iodine. Guess what? We get this primarily through our diet, meaning our gut has to process it. Iodine absorption varies with possible levels of SIBO. Another risk factor for our thyroids is the autoimmune response that can lead to Hashimoto's Disease. When this response is triggered (by toxins leaking out of our gut), it will cause the immune system to target our thyroid gland or its T3 producing capacities (Virili & Centanni, 2015). Both of these possible scenarios lead to a condition called hypothyroidism. This disease causes a reduced capacity in the production of T3 hormones.

The signs that we must keep an eye out for in these scenarios are closely related to a lack in production of T3 and, therefore, ATP energy. We are, of course, talking about chronic fatigue, but with it comes depression as well. The metabolic processes will be slowed down with additional warning signs including constipation or unexpected weight-gain. Less obvious signs would be that of dry skin and thinning, dry hair due to a lack of certain oils required for homeostasis. Though we should know this by now, our diet is going to determine our energy levels. This is, therefore, even more of a reason to ensure our gut health is as optimal as we can make it.

7. EMOTIONAL DISTURBANCES

As I have been mentioning in previous sections, we may be able to notice a pattern by now, a connection between the diseases being described. That is why, if we want to tackle our health in a holistic manner, we must take the whole picture into consideration. Our brain, and hence our mental state, is not exempt. The systems between our gut and brain are mediated by neuroimmune, neuroendocrine, and sensory pathways (Winter et al., 2018). By now, the relationship between the gut microbiome and depression is well-documented and has been verified time and again. The same goes for anxiety. These are going to be the two main warning signs we will go over in this section.

In this epoch of comfort, you would think depression levels should be going down. We need only press a button in order to have a meal delivered to our home. We can stay in touch with all our loved ones, no matter how far away they are.

Yet, suicide and depression levels are on a steep rise, and have been for quite some time. Pinning down a single causal factor to this epidemic is quite difficult because, as previously stated, everything is interconnected. In fact, both social and biological factors must be addressed in order to come to any sort of conclusion.

What we can say for certain is what the evidence and research have provided us. There is a connection between the diversity in a person's microflora and major depressive disorder. This means that an important factor may very well be the way we are eating and what sort of chemicals we are being exposed to. To be precise, the increase we are seeing in depression was eighteen percent between 2005 and 2015. There are more than 300 million people reported with depression currently (WHO as cited in Winter et al., 2018). Depression enfeebles our immune system in a way comparable to the way people affected by HIV are weakened. As mentioned by Walker, "Recent meta-analytic data indicates that people with depression have a relative risk of mortality from all causes that is 1.86 times that for non-depressed individuals and that there are 2.74 million deaths annually from depression" (Walker et al. as cited in Winter et al., 2015, p. 3). A good point made by Winter (2015) is that the brain does not exist in isolation, but is inherently connected with a human's overall physiology. This, of course, supports the idea of organic determinants for more subjectively perceived disturbances.

The relationship between microbiota and depressive states is a dialectical one. By this we mean a reciprocal exchange in which the combination of the two factors form a new product, creating a spiral of thesis, antithesis, and synthesis. It is a spiral because the new product or synthesis becomes the next thesis which will then be changed by a new antithesis. Depression may cause dysbiosis as much as dysbiosis can cause depression. Each condition conserves the other and helps each become more prevalent. Let's keep in mind that the communication in the brain-gut axis is bidirectional. The gut can send signals as well as receive them from the brain. Although it is bidirectional, eighty percent of the nerve fibers that carry information in the vagus nerve are afferent. This means that they carry information from the gut to the brain, and only twenty percent goes from the brain to the gut. The way these conclusions have been reached is through our germ-free mice. I do want to acknowledge the fact that germ-free mice are not equivalent to small people; however, this does open a door for clinical studies to be made. The results in recent experiments were consistent and reproducible (Winter et al., 2015).

Levels of serotonin, dopamine, and gamma amino-butyric acid (GABA) are associated with depressive symptoms in humans and mice alike. The brain and the gut can communicate directly through the vagus nerve, but indirect communication is established as well. Our gut microbiota influence the levels in which we produce and absorb the neurotransmitters associated with depressive disorders. Correlations clearly associate microbiota biodiversity to the depressive levels. The mechanism by which this happens is thought to be an excess in the production of cortisol, which is known to alter the equilibrium found in the microbiome of our gut. This is not certain and further research in the field is required to determine the mechanism, but the relationship remains clear. The trend across many studies revolves around the rise of the Actinobacteria and Proteobacteria phyla in individuals suffering from depression. Finally, in a study carried out by Zhen (as cited in Winter, 2018) microbial samples were transferred from depressed individuals into germ-free mice. The germ-free mice then went on to exhibit behavioral patterns similar to those of a depressed person.

Anxiety also influences the levels in which we produce cortisol in our bodies. Cortisol has been mentioned previously as the hormone related to stress. Uncontrolled worry or fright will inundate our bodies with unhealthy levels of cortisol. This profoundly affects our body, the gut microbiome not being an exception. Cortisol is directly tied to a decrease in microbiota diversity. If you are suffering from depression or anxiety, you may have a lack of interest in the world and a loss of motivation. Becoming aware of it is the first step to change, but awareness without insight can lead to frustration and feelings of hopelessness.

Fortunately, there is a way out, which will be discussed in great detail in the following chapters. One must first take responsibility for oneself and understand the role one has taken in one's life. From here on out, a conscious decision must be made. The path is full of obstacles, but they are obstacles we place in front of ourselves.

8. BEHAVIORAL DISTURBANCES: FOOD CRAVINGS

From time to time, you might find yourself thinking you would like to have a healthy day as far as your meals go, but throughout the day, you get this "gut feeling" that you just want a piece of cake. Perhaps you get a craving for that new hamburger you saw announced not too long ago. What if I were to tell you that those cravings are not truly your own? You are, in fact, feeding into what certain microorganisms are asking you for. These microorganisms are simply looking out for their own benefit, not necessarily yours.

One example of how microbiota can influence a mammal's behavior can be found by referring back to our germ-free mice. The specific mice used for these experiments were classified through their behavioral patterns. For example, one group of mice fell into the adventurous category, while the other fell into the timid category. Through the transference of microbes, timid mice could be changed into adventurous ones and vice versa. This shows just how efficiently microbiota can transform our behavioral patterns, for better or worse. The mechanism by which microbes are transferred is called Fecal Microbiota Transplantation (FMT). This is when the stool which includes a certain set of microbes is introduced from one subject to another. Keep in mind that this is a more drastic method of microbial transference; a more gradual method would be through our diet. Much research is still required before we are able to manipulate an individual's personality or behavioral patterns through stool transference. There are findings already pointing in this direction. Introducing gut microbiota from one subject to another is extremely dangerous. The microbiome of each individual is different, and the interactions that could occur need to be calculated. For these reasons, experimentation on human microbiomes is unethical. This will delay clinical applications to some extent, at least as far as Fecal Microbiota Transplantation goes (Synowiec et al., 2018).

We had mentioned that the vagus nerve was the canal by which most communication from the gut to the brain occurs. If for some reason this nerve's capacity to communicate messages decreases, we will notice a massive loss in our body weight due to a loss of appetite. On the other hand, if this nerve is overstimulated, it can lead to excessive eating. Gut microbes are in charge of regulating just how much this nerve is stimulated or not. Microbiota can produce large amounts of dopamine and serotonin, and these neurotransmitters are used to stimulate our pleasure receptors. They activate the reward system inherent to us. Not only can gut microbes produce these neurotransmitters, but they can also block these components from being transported. As we know, a lack of serotonin being transported or produced can lead to depression.

Microbiota influence your food preferences in order to sustain themselves. The more of a certain type of food you consume, the healthier and stronger the bacteria associated with that type will become. In turn, this makes you want more of that same type of food. Another way that microbes can influence our food preferences is by modifying the composition of our taste buds. Germ-free mice have a difference in their taste buds as compared to normal mice. The effect of this change in the mice's taste buds was that it caused them to have a sweet tooth. It increased these mice's preference toward sweets, and the amount of sweet taste receptors they had. Next time you have an unreasonable craving for an item that is not particularly good for you, ask yourself: Who am I indulging here?

9. OBESITY

This is another condition on a constant rise that is once again associated with a modern lifestyle. A decrease in physical activity along with easy access to energy-dense foods can be factors influencing the steady climb of this condition. Obesity is a multifactorial condition caused in broad terms by an unbalance between how much energy is consumed against how much energy is spent (Sanmiguel, Gupta, & Mayer, 2015). The multiple factors that lead to this state of inequality aren't fully understood yet. Studies done on germ-free mice have shown that if we introduce a certain set of microbiota into the mice, we can keep them from becoming obese. They are kept from becoming obese even while they are fed a high fat and sugar diet. Needless to say, the mice who didn't have this set of microbes did become obese. These experiments show great promise for future clinical applications in the field of obesity.

If we look back at the previous sections, we can remember that our microbiota are able to modulate our appetite as well as our food preferences. If we have a larger than usual amount of microbes that enjoy foods high in fat and low on fiber, we can only imagine the consequences this will have on our taste buds and, in the long-term, our health. Human studies carried out also yielded results aligned with the germ-free mice experiments. Obesity in adult humans was correlated with a decrease in the *Bacteroides* population and an increase in the Firmicutes phylum. It is, again, a reciprocal relationship; our diet will change the composition of our microbiome as much as our microbiome will influence our diet. All research seems to be leading the way to a future where engineering certain kinds of bacteria to prevent obesity is possible (Sanmiguel, Gupta, & Mayer, 2015).

I have insisted on the fact that we don't resign ourselves to be placed under a label. Let's not become the conditions we may be experiencing. I know for a fact that these ailments are reversible. We help people with these issues on a day-to-day basis. In the following chapters, we will focus on what we can do to create change in our life. One of the best ways we can create change in our microbiome (while bacteria engineering is still under development) is by changing the sort of compounds we put into our gut. We can tilt the scale in favor of the microorganisms that are there to benefit us.

CHAPTER SUMMARY

In this chapter, we've discussed nine warning signs that your gut needs healing. Specifically, we've covered the following topics:

- Food sensitivities and allergies
- Gas and bloating
- Irritable bowel diseases
- Autoimmune diseases
- Malabsorption and nutritional deficiency
- Thyroid and energy production
- Emotional disturbances
- Behavioral disturbances and food preferences
- Obesity

In the next chapter, you will learn about the top five triggering components causing poor gut health. This next chapter will help you understand why consuming certain foods can be detrimental to your overall health.

4

TOP 5 TRIGGERING COMPONENTS CAUSING POOR GUT HEALTH

1. GMOs
2. Antibiotics
3. Gluten
4. Dairy
5. Sugar

In this section, we want to talk about certain components we are exposed to in our daily lives, possibly unknowingly. These components may severely affect our microbiome's integrity, and hence our own. The order in which these next sections are presented is by no means hierarchical. Each section will have interactions with the next, so they are all equally important. These are to be avoided at all costs, and should not be a major part of our diets, no matter what warning signs you may be manifesting, if any at all.

1. GMOS (GENETICALLY MODIFIED ORGANISM)

The term GMO refers to any organism whose DNA is engineered genetically. Bacteria is the easiest to engineer. We are going to be focusing on GM foods, or genetically modified foods. These are foods that have had their DNA altered in ways that would not naturally occur through mating and reproduction. Since GM foods were introduced back in 1996, there has been a rise in chronic illnesses such as food allergies, digestive disorders, obesity, diabetes, and autism. To be precise, the rise has been from seven percent to thirteen percent in the case of autism.

Often, GMOs are produced while keeping a human's well-being in mind. They are usually made to protect crops from fungi, microbes, insects, and other living organisms while working against negatively affecting our body's cells. In most cases, GMOs won't affect our cells directly, but the microbiota's well-being is not taken into consideration. A lot of these compounds are built to eliminate microbes, and they do not discriminate between pathogens and beneficial bacteria (commensal bacteria).

One of the more popular pesticides in GM foods created by Monsanto is called glyphosate. The premise behind this pesticide is that it attacks a particular metabolic component called the Shikimate Pathway not present in mammalian cells, including human cells. Its targets are microorganisms, fungi, and plants. Glyphosate was originally used to kill weeds. The problem here lies in the fact that, even though all microorganisms produce waste in our bodies through metabolic processes, the waste produced by pathogens has adverse effects on us. Glyphosate has shown to have profound effects on our Enterococcus phyla, which antagonize and keep pathogens such as *Salmonella* and *Clostridia* at bay. Glyphosate dwindles the amount of beneficial bacteria we have and frees up resources for the pathogens to reproduce (D'Brant, 2015). To make matters worse, pathogens have grown resistant to glyphosate.

Our main goal would be to avoid these types of food, even though they may be designed to be harmless to humans, because they continue to leave our microbiota out of the equation. Organic foods rich in naturally-occurring organisms will help diversify our microbiome, consequently making us more resistant to pathogens. You can identify these through labels that say "100% Organic" or by resorting to items locally grown.

We must be careful when looking for these types of items. Marketing departments have caught on to the growing demand for healthy nutritional options. Items can be promoted as being healthy, but really just serve as a means to catch a trendy subculture's eye while not taking our well-being into consideration. It is great that more products are being produced to target conscientious human beings; we can use capitalism itself to create change through the supply and demand ideology. The problem occurs when these organizations are only looking out for themselves. It would be advisable for you to recognize genetically modified (GM) food strains. The most popular GM foods, in the United States at least, are tortilla chips, veggie burgers, tofu, soy milk, granola bars, corn cereals, and products used for baking. Companies have done a good job at positioning a lot of these products as the "healthy alternative," but we mustn't place our trust in somebody who is just out to make a buck.

This leads to a last piece of advice when steering away from GM foods. Even if the specific item you are buying is GM-free, if the item contains soy or corn, those sub-ingredients could be GM foods themselves.

2. ANTIBIOTICS

The name of this antimicrobial substance literally means "against life." It is a substance used to target specific bacterial infections, and it has saved us from several extreme situations. This should be the manner in which they are perceived: We should see them as drastic courses of action to take against severe bacterial infections. Looking to antibiotics to help us heal from any discomfort we may come across could alleviate our pain instantly, but in the long-run, we are destroying our microbial biodiversity.

It is well documented that antibiotics lead to an overall decrease of our intestinal microflora (Ferrer et al., 2017). If we have less microbial diversity, we have a weaker immune system and less protection from future pathogens. This means we will have to rely on antibiotics next time we are colonized, since our microflora will be too weak to protect us. In most cases, we really don't need to take antibiotics. Statistics show that 80 out of 100 children who take antibiotics for a health issue have healed within seven days, and 70 out of 100 children who do not take them have the exact same result. That means antibiotics only help ten percent of the population. Our microbiome does offer the colonization resistance function; sometimes we can allow our body to do the healing, which will strengthen our immune system by allowing it to recognize the way pathogens function. I like to call antibiotics a grenade bomb inside the gut. If you can avoid them at all costs, then by all means please do so.

There are natural and less intrusive compounds that can carry out antimicrobial functions. Garlic has proven to be a less drastic antimicrobial substance. It decreases the amounts of pathogenic bacteria while proving to be a prebiotic for our beneficial bacteria. Prebiotics are components that feed our existing healthy bacteria. An experiment using garlic was carried out on mice. These mice were given a high-fat diet to cause dysbiosis. The amount of pathogens had risen, but through the administration of garlic, these levels decreased. This came along with an increase in commensal or healthy bacteria. However, an excess of garlic is not advisable either, due to its antibacterial properties (Chen et al., 2019). One clove of garlic per day is the recommended amount. Oregano oil and Colloidal Silver are other alternatives that supply an antimicrobial function. Oregano oil is recommended at 500mg, or 5 drops, daily, while Colloidal Silver is recommended at 1 to 2 tablespoons per day.

The dairy and meat industries must pump their animals with painkillers and antibiotics. This is largely due to the conditions the animals are held in. Even so-called "happy" farms keep large numbers of animals crammed together in small sheds. Cages are used for the regular kinds. The animals held there can hardly move due to a lack of space, and must defecate right where they eat and sleep. Due to the large number of animals held, some die and go unnoticed for days and even weeks. The accumulation of fecal matter and animal corpses allows for pathogenic bacteria to propagate. If the animals are not given antibiotics, they will not be able to survive long in those conditions. They would succumb to infections, especially since a lot of the time they have open pressure sores from the cages or from frustrated neighbors.

Aside from supporting inhumane conditions, the consumption of these animals provides us with a lot of unnecessary antibiotics, not to mention the genetic alterations made to the animals in order to grow at accelerated rates. The excessive amount of antibiotics being given out is a major cause for concern. Pathogens are growing increasingly resistant to antibiotics because of the excessive amounts we consume. Strains of treatable common bacteria are now becoming a threat. There are certain strains of gonorrhea and tuberculosis that have grown resistant to nearly all antibiotics. By 2050, it is estimated that if change does not occur, we won't be able to treat many of the bacterial infections we have under control at the moment. The quality of the meat or dairy being consumed must be monitored. Antibiotics reduce our intestinal diversity, leaving us exposed to opportunistic pathogens.

3. GLUTEN

About a few hundred years ago, life expectancy was at roughly 35 years. Now it is in the 80s. Recently, for the first time in the last few decades, studies are showing that life expectancy has dropped for the older millennials and Generation X. This, along with an increase of autism from 1 in 5,000 to 1 in 68, supports the idea promoted by the hygiene hypothesis. The idea is that our fight against germs has been carried out effectively. In fact, it may have been too effective for our own good. We are changing our environment too quickly, and we are not giving ourselves time to adapt. The introduction of cereal into children's diets has had a similar result.

As with the other diseases related to our autoimmune responses, celiac disease has been rising steadily as well. Celiac disease is an autoimmune disorder triggered by gluten that generates damage to the small intestine. Statistically, celiac disease is now prevalent in one percent of the US population. Gluten can be found in wheat, rye, and barley products such as pastas, breads, crackers, and cereals. It is a protein whose consistency is glue-like. It provides pasta with its structural sturdiness, for example. This glue-like consistency that holds together these different foods continues being stubborn even when we ingest it. The first reason gluten isn't ideal for our gut is because of how hard it is to digest or break down the protein. When it doesn't get broken down, it's taken to the colon in its complete form, where it is then metabolized by inflammation-causing microbes. The metabolites, or the material produced by this bacteria, trigger autoimmune responses in our gut. Another issue with gluten is that it can bind or stick to proteins inside of our immune cells, which leads to an unnecessary autoimmune response as well (Berez et al., 2014).

How we react to gluten is largely determined by genetics, but environmental factors do play a large role as well. A critical moment that determines how our body is going to react to gluten is actually the first time we are exposed to it (Berez et al., 2014). At this pivotal point in our life, the constitution of our microbiome is a determining factor as to how our body will assimilate the protein. As we have discussed previously, one function of our microbiome is to train our immune system. We have to think of our gut as the primary medium with which we incorporate our environment into our body. Our body then needs to learn how to filter and possibly fight off less beneficial influences. If our immune system is trained appropriately by beneficial bacteria that stimulate it, we will become tolerant to incoming stimuli. It will raise the threshold to only be activated when under serious threat of an infection. On the other hand, if pathogens have their way, they will overstimulate the immune system and make it reject every little stimulus it gets, leading to chronic inflammation. This is how a disease or any sensitivities to gluten start. It is through repetitive damage over time that we start to even see symptoms.

How we react to gluten is affected by our microbiome's constitution at the time of ingestion. Additionally, gluten affects the way our microbiome is made up. For instance, even if you are predisposed to type 1 diabetes, the chance that you will actually manifest symptoms is a lot lower if you are to follow a gluten-free diet. The mechanism by which our microbiota protects us against diabetic disorders is still unclear, but the correlations are quite precise. This protein is by no means necessary in our nutrition. Gluten was added to our meals due to the chewy or elastic sensation it provides when ingested. Gluten sensitivity is what we may call it when we manifest discomfort after ingesting gluten, quite similar to the symptoms associated with lactose intolerance. Bloating, puffiness, gas, feeling lethargic and fatigue are the warning signs we want to look out for when it comes to these types of food.

4. DAIRY

For us to be able to imagine how dairy may impact the microorganisms in our gut, we must think about the process dairy cows go through to produce our milk. In the search for profit, the dairy industry has developed methods to increase efficiency. Increasing the dairy cows' production time and how long they can live has been done through antibiotics and painkillers. Like us, cows have their own microbiome and are prone to infections themselves, though they may possibly be able to work out on their own. Unfortunately, allowing them to work out the infection would not be efficient for dairy producers. Bovine Mastitis is the term used to refer to inflammation of the utter through microbial infections or trauma. Due to the exploitative nature of the dairy industry combined with administration of preventive probiotics, it is safe to say that the dairy cow's microbiome is damaged and ill-equipped to deal with future microbial attacks. Afterwards, when the dairy cow becomes a victim of microbial colonization, it would now have to rely on antibiotics once more. Infections in dairy cows are so common that there is an allowed level of pus permitted by each country's state in the milk produced. In the US, for example, over 500 million pus cells per liter are considered an adequate level in the milk we drink.

There are a few conclusions we may draw about how this can affect us. The dairy cows must be in a state of dysbiosis, sheltering a larger amount of inflammation-causing bacteria because their intestinal flora has been flushed since they were young through the use of preventive antibiotics. We have already seen the effects of flushing a mammal's intestinal flora in mice. It makes their immune system weak, so they can't fight off pathogens and become reliant on antibiotics. When we ingest this pus-filled milk, we are exposing ourselves to a beverage high in the wrong types of microorganisms. Now, in ideal circumstances, dairy actually provides a healthy diversity of microorganisms for us, which is why fermented dairy is considered a probiotic. With the propensity these animals have to infection, we are really taking our chances here. The second factor to look out for would be the residue left from the probiotics possibly administered. Are we to trust people who are just out for a profit? It's a bit of a gamble; there are other sources of food which are much more reliable, as well as free of suffering and enslavement.

5. SUGAR

Historically, sugar used to be extracted from sugarcane, and was mainly used for medicinal purposes and as an item exclusive to nobility. Times went on, and through the use of slavery, the cost of sugar went down and became a staple in the working-class man's diet. About one hundred years ago, the average amount of added sugars Americans would consume daily was 62 grams. Now this number has risen to 100 grams, on average, per person, daily. This is four times the recommended amount.

This tendency to seek sugar has been programmed into the reward systems of our brain. Sugar preference at one point in time helped us survive, allowing us to distinguish edible fruits from other less-favorable ones. This sugar preference has long outlived its usefulness as a biological trait within us; it is no longer adaptive. The change in the amount and type of more prevalent chemicals in our gut is going to change the type of microorganisms that flourish (Rienzi et al., 2020).

When we are thinking about our microbiome, let's avoid looking at it as a homogenous, unified entity. The microbiome has its similarities to the way we inhabit Earth. There is geography to it, meaning that certain communities inhabit different locations of our gut. These locations are referred to as niches. The microorganisms will flourish where there is less competition for their required nutrients. Increasing the levels of sugar in our diet allows for pathogens to create more communities and reduce the diversity in our gut. Additionally, normally beneficial bacteria also begin to adapt to the high-sugar diet we have been providing them with, causing them to become pathobionts. Pathobionts metabolize the sugars in our gut and turn them into less-than-beneficial inflammation-causing byproducts. This is especially the case when we reduce the amount of fiber we consume. If our commensal bacteria do not have the nutrients they need, they will adapt and move on to use what you are providing them. This is why we must ensure they have enough of the right type of nutrients (Rinezi et al., 2020).

Even worse than sugar is another substance that goes by many names. You may come across refined sugar variants such as corn syrup, high fructose corn syrup, glucose syrup, natural fructose syrup, corn sugar, and many more titles that implicitly suggest their "natural" origin. This elusive name-changing is an attempt to avoid the recent attention high fructose corn syrup has been receiving from the nutritional community. The trendy low-fat diets that kicked in have caused an enormous increase in the consumption of sugar. As we will see shortly, a low-fat, high-carb diet is exactly what has brought about the epidemic of obesity and gastrointestinal diseases (DiNicolantonio & Berger, 2016).

Among all the sugars, however, high fructose corn syrup is by far the worst. It is mainly due to the extremely large amount of fructose present in this item. You may think to yourself, "But isn't that the sugar fruits contain?" The answer would be yes, it is, but fructose is present at much smaller amounts in fruit. The fructose-to-fiber ratio you ingest from most fruit is actually quite good for you. You would have to eat a massive amount of fruit for fructose to be an issue. It is said that the difference between medicine and poison is the dose. This is precisely the issue with high fructose corn syrup; it is poison in the amount that is present in most of our foods. High fructose is present in unnatural and unhealthy amounts in our food. Additionally, these refined sugars negate the satiety effects our body is supposed to send to our brain. Leptin, which is the satiety hormone normally produced in our gut, is not produced, and therefore we may consume all the corn syrup we want without feeling full. We may consume an extremely high amount of calories, and our body won't even warn us. This is how people have become obese. It is not due to their gluttonous predisposition; it's because this poison fools people into eating more than they should. This, of course, is good for the corn syrup producers' pockets.

Poison can be referred to as a substance that our body cannot metabolize in a healthy way, leading to a buildup of harmful toxins. Some poisons act quicker than others, of course. High fructose corn syrup is identical to that of ethanol. Any effect you associate to the chronic consumption of alcohol can be associated with the ingestion of refined sugar. Let's elaborate on their similarities a little further. The only organ that can metabolize these poisons is the liver. As we know, alcohol has profound effects on the liver. Cirrhosis is probably the most famous of the outcomes of chronic alcohol abuse; it is due to years of damage and scarring in the liver. High fructose corn syrup induces the same kind of cirrhosis, except you don't even get a buzz off fructose. Just like alcohol, most of the calories taken through corn syrup are transformed and stored as the wrong type of fat and cholesterol. Corn syrup makes you twice as fat as fat would. Carbs found in crackers and white bread can be considered empty calories, which provide little nutritional value per calorie. Corn syrup does not translate into empty calories. We are talking about harmful triglyceride-raising, fat-producing, and liver-damaging calories here.

Unfortunately, reading the ingredients on foods is risky due to how sly the corn syrup producers are. Foods that contain these products are mainly processed, not foods that you would prepare at home. We don't have a bottle of corn syrup sitting around, so our best bet would be to just avoid any processed foods. This means not consuming soft drinks, potato chips, ketchup, and most sauces found in our fast food. An item may be advertised as low fat, but that just means the item doesn't have a lot of lipids in it; it can still have ingredients that are turned into harmful fat in your body. To top all this off, high amounts of fructose stimulate the growth of pathogenic microbes such as those of the *Candida* strains (DiNicolantonio & Berger, 2016). In the following chapter, we will be looking at exactly what it is that our commensal bacteria need to thrive.

CHAPTER SUMMARY

In this chapter, we've discussed five triggering components causing poor gut health in depth. Specifically, we've covered the following topics:

- GMOs - why and how they came about, and why they are harmful
- Antibiotics - what they do to our system and how we consume them through our food choices
- Gluten - what it is and why it doesn't break down along with gluten sensitivity symptoms

- Dairy - the process of the dairy industry and why we should avoid it
- Sugar - the hidden ways sugar makes it into our food and why it's poisonous to our system

In the next chapter, you will learn about the top five foods that will assist in the process of naturally healing the gut health. We will go in depth on each recommended food item with their significant benefits.

TOP 5 FOODS TO NATURALLY HEAL THE GUT

1. Coconut
2. Blueberries
3. Pineapple
4. Fermented Foods
5. Healthy Fats

The past couple of chapters have focused on the issues, but let's not dwell there for too long. Instead, let's look for a solution. Initially, we would like to provide you with a small, easy-to-remember list of items to include in your diet. Before we do this, please keep in mind a disease is caused over years, sometimes up to thirty, of repetitive damage. Bearing this in mind, we must be patient with our body through the healing process. Pace yourself and make gradual changes in order to make it a sustainable process that you won't become frustrated with and may end up ditching along the way. As with most healing processes, persistence is key. Incorporating some of the foods we are about to mention into your daily lifestyle will allow you to see drastic changes in both your mental and physical health.

It is interesting to note that in western developed countries, sixty-five percent of people who suffer from malnourishment are overweight. Malnourishment sounds like it may be related to a lack of nutrition, which it is, but the fact that people aren't getting nutrients doesn't mean they are not consuming them. The reason is either that that empty calories are being consumed or nutrients are not necessarily being absorbed. Energy is being consumed, but not produced and therefore not spent. This is where dietary fiber comes in as an alternative to our current epidemic of malnourishment.

Dietary fiber is defined as the plant matter that is not digestible by human digestive enzymes. Instead, these fibers can be digested by our microbiota. They are carbohydrates. The main ones are cellulose, which is the component that makes up the plant cell's cellular wall. Animal cells do not have these, so we cannot produce this naturally in our body, and must instead consume the cells through our diet. Pectins are another type of dietary fiber which naturally occurs in fruits and vegetables. The primary categories dietary fiber is split into are soluble and insoluble. This isn't highly relevant when we make our food choices, since in most cases if we make the right food choices, we will be consuming both types.

When we think about some of the reasons why we should increase our fiber intake, it will simply lead us back to the repercussions a low-fiber diet can have on our microbiome's diversity, and our intestinal lining. Additionally, to all the benefits we have associated with a healthy microbiome, a high-fiber diet provides us with the prevention of gastrointestinal types of cancer. Cancer is thought to be a reaction or mutation of cellular genesis brought about through continuous damage or misuse of our body's cells. At one point, the cells simply stop cooperating with the rest and become abnormal cancerous cells, which tend to reproduce and influence those around them.

Fiber-containing foods modulate our hunger/satiety hormones, allowing our body to provide us with healthy signals as to when we have consumed enough calories. If we wait twenty minutes after ingesting a portion of food, we will know if we should eat more or not. Our body will tell us through the release of leptin hormones. This is why it is important to eat slowly and really enjoy your meal. Finally, fiber does reduce the absorption of carbohydrates in our small intestine, which allows the carbs to be metabolized by the microbiota in our colon, leading to farts instead of fats. Less absorption means less sugars are transformed into fat, and instead, our bacteria causes us a little flatulence. That sounds like a pretty good deal to me.

Elements of cooperation, unity, and equilibrium are found repetitively in nature, and we are part of nature, so it only makes sense to follow these same types of patterns. Thirty grams of dietary fiber and under twenty-five grams of sugar is the consensus generally agreed to bring about equilibrium. For example, an average-sized apple contains about four grams of both soluble and insoluble fiber. This is largely what the next food recommendations are going to be based on. Higher fiber meals will keep us satiated for longer.

1. COCONUT

Coconuts serve as both an antimicrobial and a prebiotic at the same time. Coconut has been correlated with an increase of healthy strains of commensal bacteria while decreasing the amount of pathogenic bacteria present in our microbiome. Specifically, it is known to cause an unpleasant environment for *Candida* and yeast infections. *Candida* are the strains that create tiny holes in our intestinal lining. The effects of coconut lead to a healthy intestinal wall, allowing for a healthier immune system, bringing down the effects of inflammation on conditions such as arthritis and fibromyalgia. Studies on mice have been carried out in reference to the ingestion of coconut oil and have proven the aforementioned statements (Heeney et al., 2018). The effects of coconut on our body surpass our gut and include antioxidant and cholesterol-improving properties. Society has shifted our view to come to think of fats as unhealthy, but a lot of healthy fats are, in fact, much easier to digest than grains and sugars.

Coconut intake is flexible. Drinking coconut water or adding coconut directly into your meals is great, but you can also resort to coconut oil. Extra virgin coconut oil can be used to cook with, and you can also place it on your skin or hair. It can also be used as a mild version of sunscreen. If you happen to not like the taste, you can add a tablespoon of it in one of your favorite beverages. In bulletproof coffee, for example, you can exchange the butter for coconut oil.

Coconut oil is broken down quickly, and the energy it provides can be used even before the whole digestive process has concluded. This is great for that alert state of mind many of us seek in the morning. There has been a movement advocating for a change in our body's fuel source. Instead of using grains containing sugars and gluten, which are known to cause inflammation and issues associated with insulin production, we can move to healthy fats as a less damaging source of fuel instead. About sixty percent of our brain is made up of fats, and our brain loves to run off healthy fats; it doesn't use carbohydrates exclusively.

2. BLUEBERRIES

Blueberries are the number one nutrient-dense food and fruit in the world. It is one of the best foods you can eat because they are high in antioxidants. They have been shown to reduce intestinal inflammation and protect the gut. Additionally, they are also low in sugar and can be metabolized easily. Eating a handful of these for breakfast should suffice. Blueberries contain a great amount of vitamins C and K, fiber, and manganese. Many nutritionists believe that if you make only one change in your diet, it should be to add more of these!

Our microbiome changes as we age, and so the biodiversity decreases with time. This also means the thickness of our intestinal lining wears out. Blueberries, with their antioxidant properties, have been linked to a decrease in the aging process that our microbiome goes through. They also prevent the thinning out of our intestinal lining (Desjardins, 2017). Antioxidants safeguard us from the corrosion caused by metabolic processes.

Blueberries are definitely top-tier when it comes to antioxidants, but a good indicator for other fruits with these properties is their color. The darker-colored fruits are known to be far richer in antioxidants. This was mentioned by James Joseph (2003). He was one of the leading researchers in the blueberry field. Blueberries are one of the most well-researched fruits, mainly due to marketing hypes associated with Joseph's discoveries in the antioxidant field. Even though there has been a lot of marketing involved in the field of antioxidants and berries, there is some truth to the matter. It is said that the whole is larger than the sum of its parts. In this case, and for some reason not yet well discerned, a whole blueberry is still found to be much more beneficial than any antioxidant supplement you may find. Not even attempts to extract a blueberry's components have met the mark.

3. PINEAPPLE

Pineapples are a strong prebiotic that help feed our commensal bacteria and tilt the scale of the bacterial war in our favor. On top of this, they contribute a healthy amount of dietary fiber. Pineapples also contains a digestive enzyme called bromelain, and it has some of the most powerful and natural anti-inflammatory compounds out there, which make pineapples regarded as one of the most anti-inflammatory foods in nature. I like to add this fruit to the list because when we are starting out in our healing process from time to time, the bugs in our gut may still have a lot of control over our cravings, and unwarranted cravings for sweets may arise. Pineapples are a great option to divert any sugar craving while still doing right by your microbiome (Campos et al., 2020).

In a cup of raw pineapple chunks, you may find about 2.3 grams of insoluble dietary fiber. This insoluble fiber is not digested by the human body, but it is instead fermented by bacteria in our gut. The metabolic products released have antioxidant effects on our body. Our symbiotic relationship with our gut bacteria really shines in this fact; we feed them with fiber-rich foods, and they slow down our aging process for us.

4. FERMENTED FOODS

Fermentation, specifically when it is done to vegetables and fruit, is carried out by microorganisms' metabolic processes. Microbes take the compounds found in our food products and make them more readily available to our body. To be precise, sugars are found in the items being fermented and transformed into more beneficial acids and peptides by the probiotics possibly present. In addition to creating beneficial substances in our foods, they can also neutralize some of the more toxic compounds such as phytic acid and unpleasant tasting phenolic compounds (Bell et al., 2018). The microbes present in fermented products themselves act as powerful probiotics. The ingestion of the microorganisms found specifically in fermented fruits and veggies expose our gut to a wider range of microorganisms, keeping our microflora diverse and balanced.

Fermentation is not a new discovery; it has been going on since ancient times. Dairy was the most commonly fermented food due to its short shelf-life. This process has been a commonplace practice throughout many cultures, including Korea with their kimchi, India's chutneys, and, of course, the European sauerkraut. Increasing the food's shelf-life was the initial reason these methods became a staple part of our cultures, and this still remains a great benefit of this type of food.

We want to stress the importance of focusing on fermented vegetables and fruits. There are other fermented products such as beer and wine, but in most cases, these undergo procedures to have microorganisms removed. Fermented wheat products go through a heating process that renders the microbes inactive. In general, it has been found that fermented fruits and vegetables are by far the best way to consume probiotics. The development of supplements hasn't reached the efficiency levels with which fermented foods increase our microflora. This may be due to the fact that probiotics are found in their natural habitat in fermented foods, and that they have the chance to interact with other microorganisms, improving each other's metabolic processes. The isolation of certain beneficial strands put into probiotic supplements hardly takes into account these possible interactions that are supposed to naturally occur. That is not to say that supplements are not effective; we are just saying that more research with a holistic tendency is required to completely understand what is in fermented foods that make them so powerful (Bell et al., 2018).

5. HEALTHY FATS

Our body can resort to either sugars, proteins, or fats for its fuel. Fat is a longer-lasting fuel than sugar, which is metabolized much quicker. Meanwhile, fat burns for longer and provides us with more sustained energy. It is safe to say that fat is twice as energy dense as carbohydrates or proteins, meaning it includes more calories per gram of fat. Metabolizing healthy fats provides fewer damaging byproducts as compared to carbohydrates. As part of the requirement for any recommendations made in this section, healthy fats do contribute to a balanced microbiome.

In general, we are talking about unsaturated fat, which does not solidify at room temperature. All those white creamy fats that harden at room temperature are saturated fats, which increase your blood cholesterol. Unsaturated fats remain closer to a liquid state at room temperature. Some examples of healthy fats are those contained in avocados, nut butters, olives and their oils, omega 3s and 6s, coconut oil, eggs, and dark chocolate. These fats' nutrient/calorie ratios are ideal, and will help you avoid malnourishment through the consumption of empty calories. A fruit that can be pointed out here is the avocado. Unlike other fruit, it is rich in healthy fats and low on sugars. It does contain an enormous amount of dietary fiber as well. The best part of it is the meat right around the edges, close to the skin. Nutrients concentrate in that area, which is why we should peel our avocados with our hands.

The second area to highlight isn't quite so popular, however. South American indigenous cultures have been using the avocado pit or seed for centuries as a way to treat gastrointestinal diseases. This is due to the fact that the seed is particularly high in polyphenols. Studies on the effects of these polyphenols have shown that they help reduce the pathogenic bacteria numbers in our gut (Signh et al., 2017). The seed has been described to have a bitter taste, or in some cases, a taste similar to that of certain types of nuts. Recommended ingestion options can be to grind it up into powder, at which point it can be placed into a smoothie, a salad, or it can even be made into tea. As a result, the properties will remain active. The combination of polyphenols, fibers, healthy fats, and antioxidants makes this fruit stand out.

When we mention omega-3s and omega-6s, we are mainly talking about fats that come from fish oils and plants. Omega-3s mainly come from fish, while omega-6s come from plant-based oils. The recommendation isn't as intuitive for the consumption ratio of these two. Omega-3s are to be prioritized over Omega-6s. These are usually issued out in the form of supplements, but they can be ingested through certain kinds of fish in our diet as well. Supplements are synthetic options that do not include animal products. These supplements are among the most popular recommendations a nutritionist or physician may make. Research shows that through maintaining the integrity of our cells, since all our cells' membranes are made up of lipids, fish oil has shown to have profound effects in the maintenance of our brain function. This is especially recommended for our aging process and has proven to protect us against disorders such as dementia.

Another association that has been made is between omega-3s and their anti-inflammatory effects on victims of arthritis. This may be partially due to the fact that healthy fats help maintain the integrity of our intestinal lining by promoting a smooth digestive process, making our gut less prone to leaking toxins into our joints.

When it comes to cooking, coconut oil, avocado oil, and olive oil are going to be the best bet. It is said that it is a better idea to spray your oils instead of pouring them: Just because we use these unsaturated fats which have been branded as healthy doesn't mean we get to go wild on them. Moderation is still required, just like too much of a good thing is still too much. Let's keep this in mind when using oil for cooking. We do want to avoid vegetable oil, since the name "vegetable oil" is vague, and it is a product developed for cost efficiency. Anything you can do with vegetable oil, you can do better with alternative oils. Besides the fact that they are healthier, they taste better, too.

Our microbiome has been receiving quite a lot of interest on behalf of the scientific community and the medical-nutritional industries. Following the extensive amount of research that has been done on the topic of microbiota, results have surged. Effective supplements that have been engineered are becoming more efficient every year. In the following chapter, we will summarize the most effective supplements you may use to complement your diet.

CHAPTER SUMMARY

In this chapter, we've discussed five of the top foods that contribute to a natural healing of the gut. Specifically, we've covered the following topics:

- The importance of fiber and its major benefits
- Coconut - its benefits and the different ways you can consume it
- Blueberries - their outrageous amount of antioxidant properties and the benefits that contribute to the health of the lining of the gut
- Pineapple - the great alternative to sugar while providing a natural prebiotic and digestive enzyme
- Fermented foods - the natural source of probiotics and the importance of consuming fermented fruits and vegetables
- Healthy fats - consuming unsaturated fats for fuel and for a balanced microbiome. We also covered some of the different sources of these healthy fats.

In the next chapter, you will learn about the top five supplements that will help heal the gut naturally. This next chapter will go over each recommended supplement with their significant benefits.

TOP 5 SUPPLEMENTS TO NATURALLY HEAL THE GUT

1. Probiotics
2. Digestive Enzymes
3. Fiber
4. L. Glutamine
5. Antifungals

In the following chapter, we will briefly review some alternative options that may be explored in order to strengthen some possibly weak areas in our nutritional routines. Perhaps you don't have access to fish very often, or can't stand the taste of unsweetened yogurt, for example. Supplements can definitely fill those gaps. These items are engineered to take efficiency and practicality into consideration. You get to obtain the nutrients you are looking for at a low caloric cost, not to mention a possibly low economic cost as well. The doses are provided in a strict fashion, which adds to the practicality of the approach. You may not know how much of what type of fish you need to consume in order to meet a recommended amount of 500mg of omega-3. However, like in the case of fish oils, supplements are not going to do you any harm in any scenario. The fish protein is usually removed, which means it will not trigger any allergies. If you can afford a supplement, then it should be taken; there is no reason not to.

1. PROBIOTICS

We have been using the term probiotics loosely throughout our different discussions. What we are referring to here are engineered sets of probiotics cultured specifically for the human microbiome. We have an understanding that there are commensal bacteria associated with healthy gut, brain, and immune system functions. Through the studies such as the ones we have reviewed, we have attempted to isolate strains of commensal bacteria into capsules. To make sure we are receiving quality strains, we want to look for the following phyla: *Bifidobacterium, Lactobacillus* and *Saccharomyces*. Let's keep in mind that these are living organisms. When we receive them, we should keep our probiotics refrigerated and dry. Moisture can activate the probiotics, and once active, these organisms will die due to a lack of nutrients. They are sensitive to heat as well, so make sure they are always stored in a cool and dry area.

Probiotics help your gut heal itself by increasing its biodiversity. It is a gradual change that occurs over time. They can target a range of microbial niches starting from our stomach and downstream all the way to our colon. Any benefits reaped in the upper regions of our intestinal tract will provide changes downstream as well. Changing the gut microbiome's constitution can help increase the water mass and consistency of your stools, consequently alleviating any strain in the anal cavity that may lead to hemorrhoids.

As we have mentioned before, probiotics are included in our meals, but due to our differing lifestyles, we may not have the time to ferment cabbage and might prefer a more practical option. Marketing has not missed a beat in taking advantage of scientific findings in the field of probiotics to make some profit. Along with the antioxidants craze, probiotics are also used by the food industry as a selling point for their products. Unfortunately, the amount of probiotics in the foods advertised is inconsequential. Let's take yogurt for example: It is probably the most popular item marketed as being rich in probiotics. In order to match the amount of probiotics you can get from a supplement using yogurt, you would have to ingest massive amounts of yogurt. This would defeat the purpose, since you would create dysbiosis in your gut through excessive consumption of saturated fats and sugar. This is especially trye for sugar, since most brands of yogurt are high in refined sugars. A healthy portion of yogurt, on the other hand, would provide a miniscule amount of probiotics, nowhere near the necessary amount to cause an impact on your microbiome.

This is exactly why supplements exist, to make it easier to target specific benefits you may need without the added side-effects.

2. DIGESTIVE ENZYMES

We can also take the proteins that break down our foods as supplements. Normally, these enzymes are synthesized when a hormonal signal is received that is usually triggered by smells or tastes. The majority of digestive enzymes are synthesized in our pancreas and salivary glands. The fact that they are synthesized in response to our taste buds demonstrates that how we eat is just as important as what we eat. If we eat too fast, our body won't have the time to produce an adequate amount of enzymes to break down the specific types of food being ingested. Our enzymes require that our small intestine displays a certain level of pH. That is the role of our pancreas; it produces a substance called bile that is introduced to the small intestine. Bile contains the digestive enzymes, along with pancreatic juices, which adjust the pH levels.

Digestive enzymes act as catalysts by breaking down complex molecules into simpler ones, increasing nutrient availability in our gut. This is opposed to allowing partially-digested components to reach our colon, where they will be fermented by bacteria. The byproducts of this fermentation can lead to flatulence, bloating, and inflammation. We don't naturally make a lot of certain enzymes, if any at all. As we age, the amount of lactase produced by the body is reduced, for example. Our genetic constitution can make it so some of us don't produce a lot of DPP-IV, which is the enzyme responsible for breaking down gluten (Taga et al., 2017). Taking digestive enzymes as a supplement before a meal can increase the amount of nutrients you receive from it and alleviate any unpleasant side-effects caused through bacterial fermentation.

These types of supplements are a good option once you have identified what type of food you are having trouble digesting. It may be that you are lactose intolerant or gluten intolerant; that is something you need to first find out through a procedure we will later explain. If you are lactose intolerant, you can take supplements that include lactase. There are more general supplements that contain a small amount of each type of enzymatic protein. If you are feeling bloated or gassy after eating a certain type of food, chances are that you are having trouble breaking this food down. In these cases, digestive enzymes are recommended.

3. FIBER

We have mentioned the benefits associated with fiber, so if you are not getting enough of it in your diet, there are supplements that can provide it. We should be ingesting about 25 to 30 grams of fiber daily, when in reality most people are only getting about 15 grams daily. Fiber can be looked at as the structurally harder parts of plant-based foods. If you have to bite into it and it's hard, then it probably contains fiber.

To get things into perspective, an apple contains about four grams of fiber, while a typical beef burger contains less than one gram, if any at all. You do want to eat the skin of fruits since that is where you will find most of the fiber. Other great sources are sturdier legumes, leafy veggies, and beans. When it comes to beans, lentils are easier to digest than most and offer about 8 grams worth of fiber per 100 calories. Calorie intake from a typical burger is from 250 to 400 per serving while providing virtually no fiber. Without fiber, you are prone to absorb all the carbs into your liver and turn them into fat cells. For one reason or another, if you are finding that you may not be getting 25 to 30 grams of fiber per day in your diet, a supplement may be a good idea, at least while you change your eating habits and preferences. Remember, our gut bacteria influence what food tastes like to us, and the intensity with which we crave it. It is understandable that change won't come immediately. We should avoid feeling guilty for our food choices and instead be grateful to ourselves for waking up and choosing to make a change.

4. L. GLUTAMINE

The amount of this essential amino acid in our body correlates with our intestinal wall's integrity. L. Glutamine stimulates the proliferation of epithelial cells, which are renewed every five to six days and require the presence of this amino acid in order to ensure top quality cells and prevent over-permeability (Kim & Kim, 2017). Individuals suffering from joint pain or chronic fatigue should think about taking this type of supplement. Even if the joint pain is not caused by a leaky gut, which in most cases it is, a leaky gut would only exacerbate the pain felt. Like we mentioned previously, a constant over-stimulation of our autoimmune system will lead to fatigue. Appropriate L. Glutamine levels will expedite the epithelial cell cycles, allowing high quality cells to be available when they are needed. People with indicators of irritable bowel syndrome or Crohn's disease show low levels of L. Glutamine, and may be candidates to take this type of supplementation as well.

5. ANTIFUNGALS

Due to the use of antibiotics or degenerative diseases, our immune systems have weakened in recent years. This has made way for an increase in the amount of opportunistic fungi that succeed in colonizing us. For years, our body has been able to fight off most of these strains, *Candida albicans* included. Consequently, our fanaticism toward synthetic antifungals and antibiotics has turned us away from the less intrusive natural alternatives. Oregano oil has been used since ancient Greek times. Aristotle is said to have noticed how a tortoise would eat oregano after it ate a poisonous snake. Therefore, Hippocrates, who is be known as the father of medicine, also advocated for the use of oregano oil to alleviate gastrointestinal issues (D'agostino et al., 2010).

Antifungals look to tilt the scale in favor of our more benevolent bacteria. These components make it so our gut bacteria don't have to battle so fiercely. These chemicals themselves create an unpleasant environment for pathogenic strains of microorganisms. Specifically, oregano oil has shown to decrease the population size of *E. coli* found in our small intestine (Zou, et al., 2016). Among the supplements in capsule form that I regularly recommend are oregano oil, walnut, and cloves. For more natural versions that you may include into your meals, you can try cinnamon, coconut oil, garlic, and ginger. At moderate doses, these can be added to your food and drink to steer away less benign microorganisms.

it is important to remember that *supplement* is a word which means to enhance another element. What we are enhancing is the balanced food choices we make day to day. We need to be conscious of what we are putting into our body and not let fighting pleasures get the best of us. With time, and through persistence, we will come to find pleasure in healthier alternatives, since our taste buds will change along with our microbial population. In the following chapter, I will share with you an efficient method that I have developed and improved with interdisciplinary help. It is a procedure to follow in order to take control of your brain/gut and regain authority over yourself once more.

CHAPTER SUMMARY

In this chapter, we've discussed five of the top supplements that contribute to a natural healing of the gut. Specifically, we've covered the following topics:

- Probiotics, including their importance and the different recommended strains
- Digestive enzymes, including when they should be taken and the benefits of supplementing them with different enzymes
- Fiber, including the amount you should consume each day and why it's crucial to having enough to heal gut health
- L. Glutamine, including what this essential amino acid does for the integrity of the intestinal walls
- Antifungals, including how powerful natural antifungals are for the good bacteria in the gut and the different antifungals that should be considered over antibiotics

In the next chapter, you will learn about the four steps, also known as the 4 Rs, to naturally heal gut health. We will go in depth on each recommended step that will help you achieve a smooth transition and contribute to a healthier lifestyle for lasting results.

4 SIMPLE STEPS TO HEAL YOUR GUT

1. Remove
2. Replace
3. Repair
4. Rebalance

These are known as the 4 Rs, and will help us achieve a smooth transition in our current lifestyle. They don't have to be followed in the order presented above. Eating a healthy variety of non-processed foods will program your microbiome to work for you instead of against you. The more diverse your diet is, the more resilient and dynamic your microbiome becomes, allowing you to enjoy the occasional treat. We are not preaching to remove all pleasure brought about by food, but equilibrium is necessary to prevent dysbiosis and discomfort.

STEP 1–REMOVE HARMFUL FACTORS & FOOD

Eventually, when these steps are followed, our capacity to find pleasure in healthier foods will increase as well. If you already enjoy the taste of vegetables and leafy greens, then this process should not be too difficult for you.

Not everybody's taste buds are configured the same way, though, and there are those of us who can't stand the taste of broccoli. Broccoli's texture is fairly crunchy if you were to eat it raw, and that is due to the high amount of fiber it contains. If you can't find a way to eat certain types of foods without bathing them in cheese or ranch dressing, then it may be a good idea to drink them instead. instead of juicing them, maybe blend them or put them through a processor. We want to conserve the pulp, which is where the fiber is. Do not strain your drink. In drinks, it is far easier to mask flavors you do not particularly enjoy, at least in the beginning while your taste buds' configuration changes. On the other hand, you don't necessarily have to consume every vegetable. You can try different ones until you find the ones you enjoy, but make sure you do your research and consume varied types. At least one of each color should provide a good variety, since the pigmentation of a veggie does provide clues to their nutritional properties. There is extensive literature on this matter. Here are some of our recommendations:

- Radishes

- Artichokes
- Leeks
- Asparagus
- Carrots
- Garlic
- Turmeric

Here are some healthy fats:

- Coconut Oil
- Flax Oil
- Olive Oil
- Avocado Oil
- Avocados
- Nuts & Seeds

The incorporation of these healthy fats will increase our brain function. You will find focusing much easier and have a more awake state of mind. By now you may have noticed that we switched the first two Rs. Usually, this method is taught as remove first and replace second, but instead, I provided you with some food suggestions which would normally be done on replace. I find that adding more of these healthy alternatives to your life helps in making the first step occur far more smoothly. As you start exploring and discovering alternatives to your current food choices, it will be much easier to remove more processed foods. The first thirty days will be the most challenging part as you fight your body's cravings and the possible addictions to gluten and sugar that have developed. The chewy texture gluten brings is something we become accustomed to, and sometimes we have a hard time identifying a meal as pleasurable without it. Fiber can replace this sensation.

When it comes to removing foods, we recommend shopping around the perimeter of the grocery stores. We must avoid the middle aisles where you will find most of the boxed, canned, and processed carbohydrates. Keep in mind the top five foods we mentioned that should be avoided. We talked about any foods containing antibiotics, such as most conventional dairy and meat products, and foods that have been genetically modified to include pesticides, meaning that we will be looking for organic alternatives. By all means, if you have your own happy cow, go ahead and drink her milk if you are not lactose intolerant. All in moderation, of course.

Gluten will not help the healing process even if you are not intolerant to it. Its sticky nature will still hinder the recovery of your intestinal lining and provide pathogenic bacteria food to thrive on. Along with gluten, refined sugar is among the most addictive items and may prove the hardest to remove. Some people simply can't bear the idea of a meal without a little white bread or some French fries. At an equal level, some people can't even think about drinking their juice without added sugar. I can safely say that a craving for some garlic bread, pizza, or pasta is fairly common, and even worse, a craving for a donut, which includes both high fructose corn syrup and gluten. As with any addiction, withdrawal symptoms will be difficult to deal with. When it comes to these symptoms, temptation is a key factor to keep in mind. It is healthier and easier for us to simply not be tempted. A good idea would be for us to create an environment where these items are not easily accessible. If you have donuts in your pantry, then you will be spending your willpower and energy resisting temptation. This constant act of resisting is tiring for our mind, and when we become tired, especially in a moment of stress or anxiety, we may very well give in. That is why, while we are reprogramming our brain and our taste buds to find pleasure in other alternatives, we should just eliminate the temptations as much as possible.

Fruits will help with our addiction to sugar, but we have to cleanse our taste buds in order to reprogram them. They have lost most of their sensitivity due to the large amounts of sugar most processed foods contain. If we eliminate refined sugars, we will be able to enjoy much subtler tastes, such as the sugar found in nature, which is present at healthy levels. Identifying products with refined sugars on them can be quite difficult. A good rule of thumb would be that if you can't pronounce an ingredient, or if there are more than five or six ingredients in the item, it is probably not a good choice. If we are to remove these few items, we should be able to starve many of the pathogens that have colonized our gut, all while not killing the good ones we need for our well-being.

STEP 2—REPLACE WITH HEALING FOODS

As we mentioned in the first step, we love to encourage our clients to add healthy alternatives to their existing diet rather than jumping straight into removing the harmful ones. If you jump into removing all the harmful components, you might feel limited as far as your food choices go. This could lead to an unsustainable and unhappy diet. We wouldn't want our brain to create negative associations toward the healing process. Therefore, when replacing gluten and sugar, we should be looking for fiber and fruits. Try to look for products with three or more grams of fiber in them and less than five grams of sugar. You can have wheat, just make it whole wheat when referring to bread, cereals, and oatmeal. Foods rich in fiber are fun to chew on and also make you feel satiated for longer. The best part of fruits is that they can stifle that sweet tooth you may have but still provide you with dietary fiber.

A major recommendation to add to your diet is that of fermented foods. If you are a fan of sauerkraut or pickled veggies in general, you are in luck. One to two forks' worth of sauerkraut in the morning and perhaps some fermented carrots or pickles as a snack should be adequate amounts. If you aren't very fond of these tastes, perhaps you can try an oriental option such as miso, which is basically fermented soy beans. Usually, it is served as a miso soup. There is a more popular option as well. Kombucha has been gaining a lot of popularity. While it has a much friendlier taste due to its sweetness, we must be careful with exactly that. Some brands of kombucha can contain over twenty grams of sugar. If you have the time and patience to learn how to make it on your own, that would be the best option. Additional options for fermented foods are:

- Cabbage
- Daikon Radishes
- Cucumbers
- Carrots
- Kimchi

There are plenty of alternatives to replace meat and dairy products. When it comes to cooking, there are typically healthy fat options such as the previously mentioned olive, coconut, and avocado oils. For creaminess, we can look to coconut products. They are made up of saturated fat, but coconut products are the type of saturated fat that is actually good for you. Most items you would think about adding butter to, you could probably add coconut oil or even some kind of nut butter instead. Coconut can also take the place of milk, and almond milk is a fine choice as well. Vegans have come up with great alternatives to meat that still taste like meat. Some alternative meat patties are made out of mushrooms, lentils, cauliflower, and soya beans. That is only necessary if you can't live without the taste of meat. Just make sure they aren't fake meats with a bunch of processed ingredients.

STEP 3–REPAIR WITH SPECIFIC SUPPLEMENTS

We try to place our client's situation into perspective and, depending on your nutritional history, this step may be crucial. If you are suffering from one or more of the warning signs we spoke about previously, it means severe and chronic damage has already taken place due to years of consistent dysbiosis and inflammation. Our commensal bacteria have been losing the battle to the pathogens for quite some time now, and in order to see swift improvement, we may have to give them an extra push. Aside from removing the constant damage and poison we put into our body, we might need to take one step further to complement the changes in our diet we are making. To do this, taking supplements is important, at least while your commensal bacteria can get a good hold of things again. You may spend a little more on the supplements, but any spending done in your healing process should be looked at as an investment. If you feel better, and if you rid yourself from chronic fatigue, depression, or inflammation, your perceived motivational levels will rise. When you couple together a stable motivated state of mind with an increased absorption of nutrients which increases the levels of energy produced, we will be left with a person in control of their own body and their destiny. The benefits reaped will possibly lead to success in many areas of your life, including your economy. On the other hand, lethargic and unmotivated states can cost us our dreams. This feeling of not being able to progress is understandable when your body is in a state of constant war.

In many cases, our good bacteria have most definitely lost the war. There may be a few of them left in precarious conditions, having to resort to eating whatever is available, such as toxic sugars in most cases. They may be in such low numbers that even if we do strengthen them, there are not enough of them to be able to compete with the pathogens. That is why probiotics are so important. Probiotics introduce large amounts of bacteria back into our gut. Most of the foods in our diet serve as prebiotics, which strengthen existing commensal bacteria. Only the fermented foods actually add to their population. In a healthy gut, we don't really need probiotics, since there is a balanced microbiome where our bacteria can reproduce on their own. In the state the majority of people's guts are in, however, probiotics are most definitely essential. The change must be gradual, though. We have to take it slowly. Large amounts of probiotics in a dysbiotic gut can have repercussions. First, we begin with the change in diet, and then slowly start adding in the probiotics. Preferably, we can start with cultured fermented foods, as was mentioned in previous sections. Once we have removed the damaging foods and have been ingesting fermented foods for about thirty days, we can start adding supplements.

STEP 4–REBALANCE WITH HEALTHIER HABITS

Everybody's microbiome is different. There are certain similarities among family members, but even twins don't share the exact same microorganisms. Kissing somebody will create a change in your microbiome, as with many other environmental factors. By now, we know that there is an intimate relationship between our brain and the microorganisms in our gut, which leads to the importance of this step. We have to monitor ourselves and practice being more aware of the thoughts and emotions that arise along with our unhealthy cravings. When you get any sort of a craving, really ask yourself, why has this craving come to me at this time? Am I really hungry? Is this craving really my own? Do I really feel like I'm being controlled like a puppet and react automatically to every urge that comes to me? If we don't practice awareness and use the information we are provided, you can be sure somebody else will. That means those in charge of creating the addictive compounds in our food are aware of what they are doing and what effects these compounds have on us.

In order to gain equilibrium in your gut, our mind must enter a balanced state as well. This means not using our imagination in unproductive ways. Lingering too much in the past can lead us to melancholic states and then depression. Worrying too much about the future creates a state of anxiety. A healthy balance of reflection on the past and planning for the future while enjoying the present is highly recommended. This may sound slightly mystical, but studies do show that cortisol is produced in both of these states. Consequently, an excess of cortisol leads to questionable food choices, and increased appetite (Chao et al., 2017). We have seen people eat out of sadness, and usually the foods that are sought out are not celery sticks. It is far more common to see somebody going to town on a tub of ice cream. The studies particularly show that cortisol leads to cravings for high fat and sugar products. Ice cream is basically just frozen saturated fat and high fructose corn syrup.

We propose a relaxed state of mind to reduce cortisol levels in our body. High cortisol levels also impact our gut directly, as we mentioned in previous chapters. One of the best ways to decrease cortisol levels while reducing stress is to exercise. Exercising also helps release some of that excess energy that, when accumulated, is used to overthink and worry.

Another complement to exercising is meditating. Sometimes they can both be done at the same time, as taught by the practices of toga, tai chi, aikido, and qi gong. Many philosophies have developed ways to induce meditative states, allowing us to be more present and aware. Science has been taking an interest in these practices and has been vouching for them for quite some time now. Some styles of meditation ask us to clear our mind, to stop thinking and be present. If we sit down and try to do this, we will notice just how difficult it may be. Random thoughts come to you about the car bill that has not been paid, what can be made for dinner, and so on. Now, if we are trying not to think, and we are not bringing about these thoughts, why are they arriving against our wishes? These are the types of questions you can ask yourself during certain types of meditation. You can watch the thoughts as they come to you in order to gain deeper insight into yourself. This process will cause a state of awareness in us where we will be far more sensitized to our own mind and thus our body. When an unhealthy craving shows up, we will have the right tools to identify its origin and neutralize the unwanted invasion. Studies have shown promising results in relation to meditation, but there are many systems to choose from. Just like there are many roads to arrive at the same destination, you can choose the system that best resonates with you (Turakitwanakan, 2013).

Being in a more awake state of mind will help you become aware of different stressors that trigger you. It is essential to question and monitor yourself in order to understand why you are being triggered by these stressors, and if you should allow them control of your moods. One triggering event can cause a ripple effect into the rest of your day. It is also important not to talk or think about negative situations while you are eating. Instead, pause, breathe, and give thanks to all the plants, animals, and people who have helped create the food nourishing you and your body. It is well known that the simple state of gratitude has beneficial effects on our brain's core functions (Kini et al., 2015). There are many studies showing how negative talk during eating affects your digestion and nervous system, as well as how it's not conducive to your overall health and well-being. I do not want you to just change the food on your plate but also change the way you eat it, too. That starts with creating new mealtime habits, eating as many meals as possible at the table in a relaxed fashion. Having agreeable company and a pleasant environment is just as important as the food being ingested. Even though your schedule might be tight, that doesn't mean you can't relax for fifteen minutes and devote your attention and energy to appreciating your food. Creating healthier relationship habits with your food is crucial.

This doesn't happen overnight either. Common sense should tell you that you cannot reasonably expect to make major improvements in your health within just a week or two. Some research has shown that effectively establishing a new habit can take, on average, about two months, and for some, it may take as many as eight. So, make the best of this to help you be the best version of yourself. It's very possible, and it starts with being stronger than your own excuses! I have confidence in you, so you should as well.

CHAPTER SUMMARY

In this chapter, we've discussed the four steps to naturally heal the gut health in depth. Specifically, we've covered the following topics:

- The 4 Rs and what each R means

- Removing harmful factors and foods with the emphasis on the replacing step to make the removing step easier
- Replacing hurtful foods with healing foods while providing some options to consider
- Repairing the gut with specific supplements and why this step will especially help the people who have more chronic damage to their gut's lining
- Rebalancing with healthier habits by working on mindful practices and tracking what works best for you personally, becoming more aware of yourself, and tracking the different reactions you experience during or after an event

In the next chapter, we will discuss a 30-day plan geared to assist the gut in healing.

8

30-DAY PLAN TO HEAL YOUR GUT

Essentially, what we are looking to do is a cleansing. We want to start by using the four Rs previously discussed before entering a strict style of life for thirty days. The transition is going to be slow in order to get ready to do a full elimination diet. After the sixty days are up, by no means are we jumping back into our old routine, as that is just not sustainable. We are going to give ourselves thirty days to remove and replace, and once this is done, we are moving to a 30-day elimination period.

Our diet is the first step to regain control of ourselves. Our body is easily controlled through components that release unnatural levels of dopamine in our brain. We must detach ourselves from this dopamine addiction. This is what is referred to as discipline. In other words, discipline refers to our active role in resisting our body's search for pleasure in order to obtain greater fulfillment and enduring happiness. Gaining control in what you consume will lead you to obtaining more control in other areas of your life as well.

First, you can start by engaging in the first 2 Rs, replacing and removing. Add healthier options and allow yourself to start removing the harmful ones without creating a void. This step will include familiarizing yourself with healthy alternatives to the foods you already eat. Read the ingredients on the labels and focus more on whole food choices. Incorporate more vegetables into your diet without adding tons of salt or sugar. Once you feel you have enough motivation and the right tools, that means you have completed the replacement step. At this point, it is time to progress to the 30-day elimination period. To recap, this is 30 days in which we take our time removing and replacing. It can be less, but 30 days at the most so we don't lose momentum. At any point when you feel ready, start the 30-day elimination period, where you will be strict with yourself and not give in to social pressure or any type of temptation.

Once the 30-day elimination period is concluded, you should be able to see drastic changes in the way you feel. The elimination period has two purposes: cleansing and identifying. We know our gut is constantly producing new cells, which is why change can occur so quickly. Drastic changes should be reaped sooner rather than later. On the other hand, the elimination period helps us understand what components were making us feel especially bad. At this point, what you can do is try to add a single type of food that used to be in your diet that you wish to incorporate and see how that makes you feel. We want to isolate singular components. Try adding gluten for a week, for example, and see how you feel during those days. Recording it would be best. If you want to add dairy, record how your body feels after that. Check for inflammation. Ask yourself, am I bloated? How consistent were my stools? Did I feel overly lethargic the next day? This type of monitoring is extremely important in order to identify what isn't working for your microbiome. Like we said, everybody's bacterial composition is different, so it is up to you to find out what exactly you can't tolerate. When it comes to corn syrup and added sugars, nobody can tolerate those, as that's just poison and should not even be considered an option.

Most healing practices can attest to the fact that healing usually occurs as an expansive wave that starts within each and every one of us. The saying goes, before you go out and save the world, ask yourself, have you saved yourself? Have you saved your family? Have you saved your community? The expansive healing wave of love begins with yourself, and in our case, your microbiota. Once you start caring about your microbes and yourself, the progressive attitude will become contagious. Those around you will begin to notice, and if they have any hint of self-love or awareness, they will also be influenced by this act of self-care. If you are able to get people in your household to follow along with you, it will make this sacrifice all the more endurable.

Your relationship to food will change, as will your food options. The way you think about food will change, mainly by not consuming highly addictive chemicals designed to make you crave them more. The freedom and peace received after this process is difficult to describe in words, but nonetheless we do want to place emphasis on this fact. The aim is to establish a healthy emotional relationship between ourselves and our food, as well as our body. Make each and every meal choice in a self-loving manner. This 30- to 60-day process should influence your perception of food in a lifelong fashion. Enthusiasm and just a little bit of faith will carry you a long way. Before long, you experience the changes for yourself.

30-DAY ELIMINATION PERIOD

No added sugars. All added sugars, real or artificial, are out of the question. Any type of syrup, honey, coconut sugar, agave nectar, Stevia, Splenda, Equal, NutraSweet, or Xylitol should be cut out. This may sound difficult, but the difficult part only lasts for 30 days. Make sure to read the labels, as companies do try to sneak in their sugars. Anything that ends with "-ose" is prohibited: dextrose, fructose, galactose, lactose, maltose, ribose, and sucrose, to name a few. Furthermore, if you cannot pronounce the ingredient, then don't consume it. Any form of alcohol, even for cooking, is to be avoided as well.

No grains. This includes wheat, rye, barley, oats, corn, rice, millet, bulgur, sorghum, sprouted grains, and all gluten-free pseudo-cereals like quinoa, amaranth, and buckwheat. This also includes other ways we add wheat, corn, and rice, such as bran, germ, starch, and so on. Read your labels, read your labels, and get really good at reading your labels.

No legumes. This includes beans of all kinds: black, red, pinto, navy, white, kidney, lima, fava, peas, chickpeas, lentils, and peanuts. This means no peanut butter either.

No dairy or junk food. Some specific foods are a huge NO! Pancakes, waffles, bread, tortillas, biscuits, muffins, cupcakes, cookies, brownies, pizza crust, cereal, ice cream, chips, and French fries. You will notice a recommendation of ghee bliss balls, which calls for clarified butter known as ghee. This is the only dairy accepted, as it contains many healing and culinary properties that plain butter does not.

For foods that are not on this list, please use your best judgment. Focus on whole foods rather than purchased processed foods. If you must purchase an item, make sure it has only five to seven pronounceable ingredients. When in doubt, do not consume the item.

Consumable Foods: We will look at the exceptions of what we may consume. Ghee or clarified butter would be the only types of dairy we can recommend. Certain legumes, such as green beans, sugar snap peas, and snow peas are fine. While these are technically legumes, they are far closer to a pod than a bean, and green plant matter is always good for you. Vinegar in all its forms, including white and red, balsamic, and apple cider, are all okay to have. Coconut aminos and Himalayan salt are great as well.

Breakfast: A scramble of grass-fed (high-quality) meat and cooked vegetables, a cup of homemade bone broth, some fermented vegetables, and supplements.

Lunch: A huge salad with leftover protein (high-quality/grass-fed meat, offal, or fish) and a small piece of fruit, a cup of bone broth, fermented water kefir, or kombucha and olives.

Dinner: A stir-fry with some type of protein (high-quality/grass-fed meat, offal, seafood) with a lot of vegetables and allowed spices. One cup of healthy starch like cooked winter squash, pumpkin, etc.

In the following chapter, I will include more specific recipes to help you through the process. Again, let's keep in mind this is not a permanent diet; we are doing this for cleansing and identification. We need to figure out what exactly is causing our issues by slowly adding components back into our diet and, at the same time, change our emotional relationship to food.

CHAPTER SUMMARY

In this chapter, we've discussed a 30-day plan to implement for healing the gut. Specifically, we've covered the following topics:

- The 30-day elimination period and what that comprises
- Foods to avoid
- Consumable foods
- Reintroducing foods at a slow pace while tracking symptoms and feelings

In the next chapter, we will provide you with meal and snack options to assist you in your journey to heal the gut for better brain function.

9

MEAL AND SNACK OPTIONS

MORNING MEAL OPTIONS:

- 3 scoops of Farmhouse cultured kraut or kimchi
- 3-6 eggs cooked with coconut oil and herbs and artichokes
- Bowl of pineapples, blueberries and/or strawberries with coconut yogurt, cashew nuts, sunflower seeds (I usually like to add an organic high-quality vitamin, green powder, or cacao powder in this, too)
- Veggies with avocado or artichokes, bell peppers, broccoli, zucchini
- Sauteed veggies and eggs (if you must have any type of bread as toast after the first initial thirty days of the elimination diet, then have it be gluten-free!)
- Ghee Ball (ghee butter or 3 tablespoons of flax oil if

you prefer no dairy, combined with sesame seeds and raisins)

Ghee Bliss Balls Recipe - (Recipe makes approx. 10 balls)

Ingredients:

- 1 c toasted sesame seeds
- ½ c golden raisins
- 2 tsp ground ginger
- 2 tsp ground cumin
- 2" piece of fresh ginger, chopped fine
- 1 ½ tsp cardamom
- 2 ½ tablespoons organic ghee

Preparation: Place all ingredients in a food processor and mix together until well-blended. Roll into 1-inch balls. If the mixture is too soft after blending, put it in the fridge for a few minutes to cool it down, which should make it easier to form the balls.

Ghee is clarified butter and contains many healing and culinary properties that plain butter does not. Look for organic and grass-fed ghee.

SNACK OPTIONS:

- Chia seed pudding made with coconut milk
- Coconut yogurt and pineapple
- Raw pumpkin seeds, papaya seeds, and sunflower seeds
- Green smoothie: coconut milk, spinach, avocado, plant-based protein powder, flax seed powder, topped with hemp seeds
- 2 handfuls of nuts and seeds: macadamia nuts, walnuts, cashews, or almonds
- Sautéed veggies or veggie tray
- Gluten-free toast with avocado (after 30-day elimination period)
- Olives with gluten-free crackers (I recommend the brand Flackers, as these are grain-free and gluten-free)
- Dips: The Bitchin' Sauce or homemade guacamole.
- Applesauce with cinnamon, coconut oil, and cardamom (this should be homemade)

Applesauce Recipe Ingredients:

- 1 cup apple (cooked)
- 1 tsp ghee or coconut oil
- ¼ tsp of cinnamon

Preparation:

1. Peel, core, and thinly slice apples. Combine apples in sauce with 1/3 c of water and simmer until apples are tender, stirring frequently.
2. Mix and bring ghee or oil, cinnamon and applesauce to a simmer, stirring occasionally. Serve warm (I like to steam apples then put in a blender with the other ingredients).

LUNCH OPTIONS

- Chicken or turkey (well-cooked, made with tons of herbs); salad with kraut, olive oil/vinegar, carrot shavings, and walnuts
- Chicken or veggie patty with steamed broccoli, asparagus, green beans, peas, or carrots
- Veggie wrap on gluten-free Paleo coconut wrap (found at Trader Joes, Natural Grocers, or Amazon) with powdered herbs, olive oil and vinegar for dressing, green lettuces, onions, sprouts, pea sprouts, shaved carrots, avocado, and almond nut spread
- Sautéed veggies (lots) and avocado
- Asparagus spears on the side
- Farmhouse cultured kraut or kimchi on the side

DINNER OPTIONS:

- Vegetable soup; Boil vegetable options in water and season – carrots, kale, celery, onion, garlic
- Sautéed cauliflower with coriander, salt and pepper, coconut or avocado oil
- Farmhouse cultured kraut or kimchi on the side
- Butternut squash and vegetable soup

Vegetable Soup Recipe – Serves 6 people

Ingredients:

- 1 medium carrot
- 2 stalks of celery
- 4 cups of kale/chard
- 1 tbsp of ghee or coconut oil
- 5 cups of water
- 1 tsp grated ginger
- 1 ½ tsp Coriander powder
- 1 tsp fennel seeds
- 1 tsp turmeric
- ½ tsp cumin powder
- ½ tsp Himalayan pink salt
- 1 tbsp lemon juice

Preparation:

1. Wash all vegetables and cut them into 1cm pieces. Heat the oil in a big pot and add carrots. Sauté for 3 minutes.
2. Add coriander, fennel, turmeric, cumin, salt, and sauté for 2 minutes.
3. Add all other vegetables, ginger, and 5 cups of water, and simmer for 25 minutes.
4. Before serving, add lemon juice and mix well.

CHAPTER SUMMARY

In this chapter, we've provided you with meal and snack options to naturally heal your gut. Specifically, we've covered the following topics:

- Morning meal options
- Snack options
- Lunch options
- Dinner options

This leads us to the conclusion of the book.

CONCLUSION

An awakened state of mind can help safeguard us from the perils of unquestioned complacency. Whether our unfaltering obedience is directed at our internal impulses, or whether we are compliant to the standards held in high regard by our society, we must come to understand that we, too, may sway the course of both the macrocosm and the microcosm alike. For if we do not take matters into our own hands, we will be but as a puppet on a string, lifelessly reacting to each tug and stroke of our microbiota and our societal expectations. Before we are able to place our own actions in question, we must get to know ourselves. Awareness without insight leads us to a problem without a possible solution.

If you made your way to this book, it is because you have already acknowledged the fact that a change may be necessary.

Awareness and acceptance is the first step that brought you here. Insight is the next step. We hope we have sparked your curiosity as far as your well-being goes. A lot of what we have talked about should be common sense as far as the importance of what we eat in relation to our health. However, without proper research and education, the misinformation provided by many of the marketing campaigns can very well put us under a spell. It is not too late to make a change, and it's absolutely not too late to start loving yourself and your microbiota. This is especially true when considering that every seven to ten years, every cell in our body is replaced by new ones. We literally are not what we used to be. We can continue to reinvent ourselves and not fall victim to the prisons of arthritis, depression, obesity, and so forth. These are not life-defining labels. We can take matters into our own hands once again, and we must.

Sometimes we might have perceived our emotional states as outside of our control, and perhaps our energy levels as well. The internal struggle we perceive to make decisions of all sorts really doesn't have to be a struggle. It doesn't have to be a fight. We can get our body and our microbiota to work with us; we just have to agree to work with them as well. Even if modern life has placed us at odds with our microbes, we can step outside of the status quo and wake up.

We hope that through the dissemination of the consequences brought about by our modern epoch, a seed of doubt will be planted. A seed that will go on to grow into a tree of progress that may bear the fruits of cooperation and equilibrium. For cooperation and equilibrium are universal laws that rule our reality. There is no single aspect in life segregated from the rest. We are part of a totality. There is an old hermetic axiom which says, "As above, so below." This refers to the similarities between the composition of the universe and the composition of ourselves. It is similar to the quote found in the temple of Apollo in Delphi, "Know thyself, and thou shalt know the universe and God." We can notice the amount of equilibrium present in nature; the planets in our solar system do not go flying off at any given time. Instead, planets are bound in place by attractive and repulsive forces in perfect balance. Aspects of cooperation and balance in nature can be learned, and this should provide us with clues as to how we should operate ourselves, how we should handle the relationship we have with our microorganisms. Cooperation is key; they need us as much as we need them.

MESSAGE FROM PURETURE WITH PURETURE WELLNESS

Thank you for giving yourself an opportunity to experience a change in your life. If any questions arise, or if you simply have a comment, please feel free to contact me through the website at https://www.pureture.com/. At Pureture Wellness, my team's mission is to expand the healing process that has changed our own lives so that we may impact as many as we can. At the link provided below, you may find some of my other work and related literature on the website as well. You will also come across the coaching and training services I personally provide. I have worked with the human body for over a decade now and have been an athlete from a very young age. From nutritional coaching to fitness plan structures, or anything in between, please do not hesitate to contact us.

Cheers to optimal health and wellness!

~*Pureture*

FINAL IMPORTANT RECOMMENDATION:

If you enjoyed this book and are eager to undergo a complete and thorough process known as detoxification, then we want to recommend you consider grabbing Pureture's detoxification book if you haven't already. This book is where we will walk you through step by step to cleanse, detox, and reset each organ in a safe, thorough and proper order.

Go ahead and look for the title:

6 Optimal Steps for Detoxification & Reset: The Ultimate Plan to Cleanse & Heal All Body Organs for Lasting Results

This book has included a program that will absolutely change your life and get you on track for a lifelong lifestyle of healthy habits and staying cleansed. It has been geared to heal the gut and to also implement positive habits that will live with you forever.

THANK YOU

Finally, I'd love to say thank you for taking the time to read this book, to learn about how you can naturally heal your gut and brain to achieve a healthier life over all.

If you enjoyed this book, ***you would be an absolute legend*** if you could leave it an honest review. If you are reading this book in its print version, then you would be a greater legend if you could leave the review with a picture of the book.

Reviews will really allow more people like you and your loved ones who need help and answers on their health journey to see this book. Potential readers would highly appreciate any review the book receives. After you leave your review, I'd love to hear from you. If you send me an email showing your review, I will happily send you a special gift your way (trust me, you will love it).

You can visit the link below to leave the book a review:

https://www.amazon.com/gp/product/B08GFSK7P1

Email - pureture@pureture.com

RELEVANT LINKS

https://www.pureture.com

www.pureturewellness.com

Image Credit: Shutterstock.com